Women and AIDS Crisis

New Edition

Diane Richardson is a social psychologist and feminist who researches and writes on women and sexuality. In 1985 she was Visiting Professor at the Centre for Education and Research in Sexuality at San Francisco State University. She currently teaches in the Department of Sociological Studies at Sheffield University.

Diane Richardson has also written an American edition of this book, published in the United States as *Women and AIDS* (Methuen, 1988). Her other books include *The Theory and Practice of Homosexuality* (Routledge & Kegan Paul, 1981) and *Feminism, Motherhood and Childrearing* (Pluto Press, 1989). *A Woman's Guide to Safer Sex* will be published by Pandora Press in 1990.

Women and the AIDS Crisis
New Edition

Diane Richardson

LONDON   WELLINGTON   MELBOURNE

First published in Great Britain by Pandora Press,
an imprint of the Trade Division of Unwin Hyman Limited, 1987.
New edition published in 1989.

UNWIN HYMAN LIMITED
15–17 Broadwick Street
London, W1V 1FP

Allen & Unwin Australia Pty Ltd
8 Napier Street, North Sydney, NSW 2060, Australia

Allen & Unwin New Zealand Pty Ltd with the
Port Nicholson Press
Compusales Building, 75 Ghuznee Street, Wellington, New Zealand

British Library Cataloguing in Publication Data
Richardson, Diane
  Women and the AIDS crisis. – Rev ed.
1. AIDS
I. Title
616.9'792
ISBN 0-04-440357-7

Set in 10 on 12 point Palatino by
Computape (Pickering) Ltd, Pickering, North Yorkshire
and printed in Great Britain by
Cox & Wyman, Reading

For Libby

Contents

Acknowledgments

When Philippa Brewster, my editor, first suggested I write a book on women and AIDS I was reluctant. I knew that, for many reasons, it would be a difficult book to write. What eventually convinced me was my belief that this book might draw attention, long overdue, to what AIDS means for women and help them to get the support and the advice they need.

Now, having completed the second edition, I want to thank the many people who helped me. Special thanks to Philippa and everyone else at Pandora Press for their support. Linda Semple was also a great help in editing the first edition. I also want to thank Liz Young and Claudia Brusdeylins at Pandora, who were both tireless in their efforts to find answers to difficult questions. My additional thanks to Lisa Power of the Angel Project, London; Janet Green at the Terrence Higgins Trust; Gretchen Harris, Director of Patient Advocacy at Bellevue Hospital, New York; Dr Craig Keyes of the Bellevue Satellite AIDS Assessment Program; Dr John Martin at the School of Public Health, Columbia University; and Dr Nancy Padian at the School of Public Health, University of California, Berkeley, for reading and making comments on the manuscript. For providing information on the Australian experience of AIDS, I also want to thank my friend Dr Megan McCormack. Thanks also to Val Squire, Sylvia Parkin and Sue Lockyer for typing the manuscript.

Various organisations concerned with AIDS were helpful in providing me with information and advice. I would like to thank them, in particular the Terrence Higgins Trust, the

Haemophilia Society, Coyote, the Shanti Project and Project Aware in San Francisco, the Women's AIDS Network, Gay Men's Health Crisis and the Women and AIDS Project in New York, the San Francisco AIDS Foundation and, in Los Angeles, the Women's AIDS Project and Mothers of AIDS patients.

I would also like to thank certain people for their time and patience in answering my questions; Janet Green at the Terrence Higgins Trust, Fran Pierce at the Middlesex Hospital, Catherine Maier and Nancy Shaw at the San Francisco AIDS Foundation, Clark Taylor at the Institute for the Advanced Study of Sexuality, Judith Cohen at Project AWARE, Joanne Mantell at Gay Men's Health Crisis, Susann Gage at the L.A. Women's AIDS Project, Denise Ribble at the Community Health Project in New York, and Suki Ports of the Minority Task Force on AIDS.

Most women who are HIV antibody positive, or are caring for someone who is, are reluctant to be interviewed. For this reason I owe a very special thanks to the women I spoke to who had the courage to share their experiences. I am most grateful to them for that.

Finally, I want to thank my friends Jackie Davis, Dorothy Dixon-Barrow, Ann Watkinson and Libby Hawkins. This has been, in many ways, a difficult book to write and their practical and emotional support has helped greatly in its completion.

Sheffield
November 1988

Introduction

The first cases of AIDS were reported in 1981, in the United States. Initially it seemed to be a disease which only affected gay men. Soon, however, it became clear that other groups of people – injecting drug users, haemophiliacs – were getting it. This, and the discovery that AIDS could also result from blood transfusions, which meant that *anyone* might conceivably get it, captured the media's attention. Stories about AIDS began to appear with great frequency, and by mid-1983 AIDS hysteria had set in.

Interestingly, despite the widespread attention AIDS has received from the media, and the evidence that it can be transmitted heterosexually, most people don't really expect AIDS to affect them. If they think about it at all it is as 'the gay plague', a disease that happens to 'other' people. This is especially likely to be true of women. Yet women certainly do get AIDS. In Africa the disease is believed to have 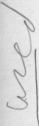 affected several thousand women, while in Europe and the United States, although the majority of people with AIDS are gay or bisexual men, a significant number of women have contracted the disease. Most of them are women who inject drugs; some are sexual partners of intravenous (IV) drug users, haemophiliacs, or bisexual men; and a smaller number are recipients of infected blood transfusions.

As AIDS becomes more widespread women who may once have seen the disease as largely confined to men are becoming more concerned about their own risks of infection. Women can no longer ignore AIDS-related problems specific to them. How can a woman practise safe sex when her male partner refuses to use condoms or have non-

penetrative sex? If she is economically and emotionally
dependent on her partner she faces a very serious conflict.
How can women who are raped or sexually abused protect
themselves from the risk of infection? Obviously, they have
been given no choice in the matter. Women not only face
problems of sexual violence but also of economic discrimination. Although the task of caring for people with AIDS
falls primarily upon women, they themselves lack support
services around AIDS and are more likely to be discrimi-
nated against in terms of receiving health care – reflecting
the low priority our society places in general on women's
health problems. Women are less likely to have medical
insurance and, in general, they earn less than men. Consequently, they are more susceptible to the financial hard-
ships which AIDS can bring. Many women are trying to
raise dependent children with little or no financial help
from the children's fathers. AIDS contracted by mother or
child can mean economic disaster for the family as a whole.
Also, there are specific problems AIDS creates only for
women; such as possible transmission during pregnancy to
the foetus.

For black women the problems are worse. In the United
States AIDS disproportionately affects the black and latino
communities. Poverty, inadequate access to health education and care, problems of racial discrimination – all put
these women's lives at greater risk. Black women's lives are
also affected by the strengthening of racist attitudes, as a
result of black people being scapegoated as the source of
AIDS. (The perception of black people as disease-ridden
and sexually 'promiscuous' is a recurring racist theme.)

This book is aimed at all women who are concerned
about AIDS, as well as the women who already have AIDS
or the virus which causes it. It is also for women who care
for people with AIDS. It provides a clear and informative
account of the issues which AIDS raises for women. In
addition to providing important information, the book also
challenges the racism, sexism and homophobia surrounding the disease.

There is so much that we still don't know or understand about AIDS that to write about it at the moment is very difficult. New discoveries are being made all the time and, consequently, some of the information in this book may need to be revised. AIDS is also difficult to write about for other reasons. It is a tragic illness. Disfiguring and debilitating to those who have it, AIDS primarily affects the young, and is ultimately fatal. Living in San Francisco during 1985 I became acutely aware of how AIDS can affect both individuals and communities. What I remember, however, is not just the sadness and the anger but also the bravery and the struggle to survive.

AIDS is not a 'gay disease'; a virus does not discriminate. It affects those who are heterosexual and gay, white and black, the wealthy and the poor, women and men, and also children. It is a social problem which we all need to be concerned about. At the same time panic and hysteria are not helpful. I hope that this book will help to remove many fears about AIDS, whilst providing women at risk with better information about how to avoid getting it.

1 What is AIDS

Acquired Immune Deficiency Syndrome or, as it is more commonly known, AIDS, is a new and fatal disease. It is thought to be caused by a virus called human immuno-deficiency virus or HIV for short. The credit for discovery of this virus is shared between French and American research-ers, although it was the team at the Pasteur Institute in Paris, led by Dr Luc Montagnier, who first announced its discovery early in 1983. The name they gave to the virus was LAV, or lymphadenopathy associated virus. The American team, led by Dr Robert Gallo, called the virus HTLV-3 or human T-cell lymphotropic virus type-3. To simplify matters researchers have now agreed to use the term HIV.

A virus is one of a group of extremely small micro-organisms that can only survive inside the cells of other living creatures. HIV attacks the body's immune system. When the immune system is impaired, the body becomes vulnerable to infections and cancers which people with intact immune systems can ward off. These illnesses are sometimes referred to as 'opportunistic infections', because they take advantage of the opportunity offered by the body's weakened immunity to do their damage. Often these infections are caused by organisms which live in everyone's body, but cause no problems as long as the immune system is not damaged.

The most common illnesses found in people with AIDS are a rare form of pneumonia known as pneumocystic carinii pneumonia (PCP), and a rare form of skin cancer called Kaposi's sarcoma (KS). It is the cancers and the opportunistic infections that cause death. This usually occurs within two to three years of being diagnosed as having AIDS. People with KS have a better chance of surviving than those with opportunistic infections. However, no one has yet been known to recover fully from AIDS.

That you can be infected with HIV and not have AIDS is something many people are confused about. In fact HIV can cause a range of conditions, of which AIDS is the worst. For example, it can lead to persistent swelling of the lymph nodes. People in whom this is the only symptom of HIV infection are said to have persistent generalised lymphadenopathy (PGL). Other people may have more serious symptoms, but still not show any signs of the opportunistic infections and cancers that are associated with AIDS. This condition is known as AIDS-related complex or ARC. It is estimated to affect up to ten times as many people as are diagnosed as having AIDS. Because it does not necessarily lead to AIDS, some prefer to use the term HIV-related illness or HIV-associated disease.

The symptoms of ARC include swollen lymph glands, severe or chronic diarrhoea, severe fatigue, rapid unexplained weight loss, drenching night sweats, fevers and yeast infections. Though it can be serious, AIDS-related complex is not necessarily fatal. Some people with ARC (an estimated 20 to 40 per cent) do, however, go on to develop AIDS.

A much larger group, some estimate as many as a hundred times the number of people with AIDS, are infected with HIV yet show no symptoms. Whether someone has been infected with HIV can be determined by the HIV antibody test. Soon after infection the body produces antibodies. Antibodies are chemical substances developed by the immune system to fight infectious agents found in the body. The HIV antibody test is a simple blood test which shows whether or not a person has antibodies to the HIV virus. It is not a test for AIDS. What it shows is whether or not a person has at some time been infected with HIV. It cannot determine whether a person has AIDS or will develop AIDS in the future.

The most common test to detect antibodies to HIV is the ELISA. (Another test, the Western blot, is more accurate but costs more and so is generally used to double-check a positive result on the ELISA). A positive test result usually means that antibodies to HIV are present, and that the virus has been in the body at some time and has caused the body to react to it. People who test positive are said to be antibody positive or sero-positive. It does not mean you have AIDS. The test does not measure infectiousness, though at present it must be assumed that anyone who is antibody positive is capable of passing the virus on to someone else who may subsequently develop AIDS.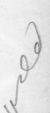

Occasionally the test produces false positives. That is, the test shows that someone has been infected when they have not. False positives tend to occur more often in women. In some cases this may be related to immune suppression following pregnancy. If your test is positive a second test is usually done to check that you do have antibodies to the virus. The results from these two tests together are very accurate.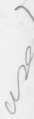

A negative test result means either that you are not infected with HIV or you have not made antibodies yet. (It does not mean you are immune to AIDS *or that you won't become infected with HIV in future*.) In a few cases no antibodies are produced though the person is infected. Also, it takes a few weeks to months after infection for the body to produce antibodies to HIV. This means that if someone were tested shortly after having been infected the test would be negative. For this reason a person would need to take the test twice, with a period of three to six months between tests, to be sure they were free from infection. During this period they should not do anything that would put them at risk of becoming infected with HIV or of infecting someone else.

There are two main aspects to the question of whether or not someone should take the test. Will knowing their test result make them more or less likely to infect others, and will it help their own physical and mental health?

If a person is extremely anxious about the possibility that they may have been infected with HIV it *may* be beneficial to have the test. Knowing that you are antibody positive also gives you a chance to alter your lifestyle in ways that may possibly reduce your risk of developing AIDS, or of transmitting the virus to someone else. This particularly applies to women who think they may be infected and are considering pregnancy (see page 58). Many people, however, feel there is little to be gained in taking the test because there is no effective treatment available for those who discover they are antibody positive, and because the advice offered is the same whether the test result is positive or negative.

If you are thinking about taking the test you should make sure that you receive proper counselling about what the test results mean, and how a positive result may affect your life, *before* you take the test. Because of the discrimination attached to being antibody positive, if you do decide to take the test you should also make sure confidentiality is guaranteed and that your results will not be put on your medical records or anywhere else. For a further discussion of the pros and cons of taking the test see pages 168–174.

Early studies suggested that about one in ten people infected with the virus went on to develop AIDS. It now seems that this figure was too low. More recent estimates – based on eight years study of the disease – are that up to 90 per cent of those who become infected with HIV will eventually develop AIDS, with some developing ARC. Because the period between infection and the appearance of symptoms is often many years, only time will show whether such estimates are correct.

Even if HIV does not affect a person's immune system, it may have other serious consequences. It seems HIV affects and damages the brain, causing a variety of psychological effects including memory loss, personality disturbance and dementia. No one knows as yet why the virus affects different people in such different ways – why one person gets pneumonia and another Kaposi's sarcoma, why one person develops AIDS without warning and another is ill for a long time before being diagnosed. Even people who have the same AIDS-related illnesses vary in the severity of symptoms.

It is also not yet possible to say what the long-term effects of HIV infection might be. No one knows how many more people who have the virus are likely to become ill in the future.

At the time of writing, the number of people estimated to be infected with HIV in the United Kingdom is about 50,000. It is vital that, healthy or not, all those who know they are infected take precautions to avoid the possibility of transmitting the virus to others. Not to do so might mean someone else's death due to AIDS.

The difficulty with this is the long incubation period. It can take anything from a few months to several years after infection with HIV for symptoms to develop. Consequently, many people who are infected with the virus don't know they are.

The kinds of precautions you should take if you are infected, or think you might be, are described later.

What causes AIDS?

The cause of AIDS is not yet fully understood. It is thought that the HIV virus must be present in the body for AIDS to occur. Although in the United States recently some researchers have questioned whether HIV is the cause of AIDS, or merely a co-factor or a symptom – an opportunistic infection which people with AIDS get. The fact that not all of those infected with the virus go on to develop AIDS suggests that other factors might be involved. Alcohol or drug use, poor nutrition, high stress levels, and frequent exposure to other diseases, especially sexually transmitted diseases, have all been suggested as possibilities. Another possible explanation is time. Recent research indicates that the chances of someone with HIV going on to develop AIDS increases, not decreases, over time.

HIV progressively undermines the immune system. It does this by attacking a particular group of white blood cells known as the T-helper cells. Normally the T-helper cells (also known as T4 cells) play a vital role in the prevention of infection. When an infection occurs they multiply rapidly, signalling to other parts of the body's immune system that an infection has occurred. As a result the body produces antibodies which attack and, hopefully, destroy harmful bacteria and viruses.

Apart from mobilising the body's defence systems to fend off an infection, the T-helper cells also signal to another group of white blood cells, known as T-suppressor or T8 cells, when it is time for the immune system to wind down its attack.

Normally we have more T-helper cells in the blood than T-suppressor cells, and when the immune system is functioning properly the ratio is about two to one. In people with AIDS that ratio is reversed, with T-suppressor cells outnumbering the T-helper cells. As a result, a person with AIDS not only has fewer helper cells available to ward off infection, but also they have an excess of suppressor cells which work against the helper cells carrying out their job.

Apart from knowing that it attacks T-helper cells we also know that, unlike most other viruses, HIV changes the structure of the cells it attacks. It does this by incorporating its own genetic code into the genetic material of the cells it infects. The result is that the infected cell is turned into a factory for producing HIV viruses which are released into the bloodstream and can infect other T-helper cells. The process is then repeated over and over again.

Viruses which function in this way are called *retroviruses*. What makes them harder to deal with than other viruses is that, because the virus becomes part and parcel of the genetic structure of the cells it infects, there is no way of getting rid of it. This means that people who are infected with the virus probably become infected for life. It also means that a person who is infected with HIV will also probably be infectious for life.

The way in which the virus destroys the function of the immune system is not fully understood. One current but unproven theory is that the destruction of the immune system that occurs in people with AIDS may be due to the body recognising its own infected T-helper cells as 'the enemy'. If this were the case, then what the body's defence mechanisms might do is start producing antibodies against the infected T-cells to try and destroy them. However, antibodies would also be produced against the *uninfected* T-helper cells, possibly destroying them as well, or making them incapable of functioning properly. In this way, HIV would destroy the immune system not simply by killing off T-cells, but by tricking the body into attacking its own defence mechanisms.

HIV doesn't only attack the body's immune system. Research has shown that the virus can also cause damage to the brain and the central nervous system. Autopsies carried out on the brains of people who have died from AIDS have revealed that the virus can cause a massive loss of brain tissue. At the same time, other researchers have managed to isolate HIV from the cerebrospinal fluid of individuals who showed no symptoms of having AIDS. These findings are extremely disturbing. Whilst researchers still thought that HIV only attacked the immune system, all those infected with the virus but with no apparent symptoms of AIDS or HIV-related illness could be considered to have had a lucky escape. Now the fear is that those who have been infected with HIV might eventually suffer damage to the brain and the central nervous system.

We don't yet fully understand all the effects HIV may have. One of the difficulties in predicting what the long-term effects of infection with HIV might be is that it is a slow-working virus. People with AIDS have been infected with HIV for some time, often for several years, before developing symptoms of the disease. As the first cases of

AIDS were only recorded in 1981, we do not know for certain what the incubation period is. It could be eight years or longer. If the incubation period is longer than has previously been estimated, then only in the next few years will the full effects of HIV become known.

Where did AIDS originate? Africa, AIDS and Racism

The simple answer is that no one knows for sure. What many people believe is that the virus which can cause AIDS probably originated in Central Africa and was exported, via Haiti, to the United States and the rest of the world. This is in spite of the fact that the vast majority of people with AIDS live in the United States. How has this arisen?

Blood tests revealing the presence of HIV-like antibodies in samples of blood going back to the early 1960s were initially cited as evidence that AIDS was common in parts of Africa before it began to appear in the United States and Europe. Yet there were no reported cases of AIDS during the 1960s and 1970s. If Africa was the source of AIDS why was the syndrome first identified in American gay men, and not in Africa? It is hard to believe that African doctors would have consistently overlooked or misinterpreted symptoms for nearly twenty years.

Scientists have also questioned the reliability of tests carried out on blood stored for many years. The longer samples are kept, the more likely it is that this will lead to false positive results.

As the theory that AIDS was an old disease of Africa became increasingly untenable, researchers put forward another explanation for the African origin of AIDS. A virus very similar to the one which causes AIDS in humans was discovered to be endemic in the African green monkey. The virus seems to have few ill-effects in green monkeys, but in a different species of monkey, macaques, it causes an immunodeficiency syndrome resembling human AIDS.

Several theories were put forward suggesting ways in which the monkey-AIDS virus could have found its way into humans. One suggestion is that the virus may have been transmitted as a result of people being bitten or scratched by green monkeys; another by eating the meat or even 'unnatural' sexual intercourse. Such ideas reflect deep-rooted racist notions that monkeys and Africans are of common descent, and are physically and evolutionary closer than people living elsewhere. Alongside this, there are other reasons which make the transmission of HIV from monkeys to Africans seem less likely. For one thing most Africans have little contact with monkeys.

The alleged incidence of AIDS in various African countries, especially in Zaire, Kenya and Uganda, has also been used as 'proof' of the African origin of HIV. According to some estimates as many as one in five people are infected with the virus in East and Central Africa. There is no doubt that the number of people with AIDS in Africa has been growing since the early 1980s, but the extent of the problem has been wildly over-estimated. According to the official statistics of the World Health Organisation, in 1987, about 10 per cent of all AIDS cases were attributed to Africa, slightly more in Europe. Over two-thirds were from the United States.

There are a number of reasons why over-diagnosis of AIDS in Africa may have occurred. It is possible that some doctors, especially those unfamiliar with tropical diseases, have confused the symptoms of AIDS with those of many other diseases common in Africa, such as tuberculosis, malaria and Kaposi's sarcoma. Also, we now know that in many cases where black Africans tested positive on the HIV antibody test, the result was wrong. (This especially applies to the more commonly used ELISA test.) This is because most Africans have been exposed to a greater range of diseases and their blood contains antibodies that can confuse the test and cause false positive results. Yet predictions about the prevalence of AIDS and HIV invection in Africa are often based on the assumption that the actual figure must be higher rather than lower than the number of cases reported.

The first cases of AIDS in Africa and North America became known roughly at the same time. If the disease originated in Africa it would seem likely that it would have spread first to Europe and not the United States, because of the closer contact between Africa and Europe than between Africa and the United States. Certainly there is no conclusive evidence linking the origin of AIDS with Africa. AIDS might have developed there but it could have equally been brought in from somewhere else.

Very little attention has been paid to theories which suggest that the virus could have originated in the West. Why? Racist stereotypes associating black people with disease and 'promiscuity' may have influenced Western researchers to over-diagnose AIDS in black Africans and to attribute them with its source. It would not be the first time that Western researchers and governments have tried to blame Africans for the origins of a harmful disease.

This is something many African governments are concerned about. Africans' concerns about being international scapegoats for the AIDS epidemic parallel those of the gay community. In the latter case the fear is that the association of AIDS with gay men will lead to renewed anti-gay and anti-lesbian feeling. In Africa the concerns are that 'blaming AIDS on blacks' will increase racism, both at home and abroad.

It is understandable that Africans should have reacted in this way. Some countries fear the economic consequences of being described as centres of HIV infection, especially in terms of how it would affect their essential tourist industries. Kenya is a case in point. After coffee exports, tourism is Kenya's most important industry for attracting money into the country.

Already the tourist industry and foreign investments in Africa are affected. The Africa AIDS myth has also been used to 'justify' racist measures against immigrants and visitors from Africa. Some countries in Europe and Asia, for example, have begun to introduce compulsory HIV anti-body testing for African visitors.

Apart from the link with Africa, there has been speculation that the AIDS epidemic is the result, either deliberate or accidental, of experiments in germ warfare carried out by the CIA. Another suggestion, supported by certain right-wing groups, is that people in the United States have been infected with the HIV virus by government agents of the Soviet Union. Others, like the Moral Majority, have claimed that AIDS is a punishment from God for society's 'acceptance' of homosexuality, promiscuity and prostitution.

How Serious is AIDS?

Any disease which invariably results in death, and for which there is no vaccine and no known cure, is extremely serious. It becomes all the more so when it spreads rapidly.

AIDS is a new disease. The first cases were seen in the late 1970s. Since then, the illness has been diagnosed around the world with increasing frequency. By November 1988 over 124,000 cases had been reported worldwide, in countries as far afield as Norway, New Zealand and Brazil. The World Health Organisation estimates that the real figure might be at least double that, since many cases go unreported. In the United States alone there are over 75,000 recorded cases (October 1988), whereas in Australia, where the first case of AIDS was reported in 1983, 943 people have been diagnosed with the disease (August 1988).

The number of new cases of AIDS continues to grow. In the United Kingdom the first case of AIDS was reported at the end of 1981. Since then the number of cases reported has increased rapidly. For example, at the end of 1983 there were only 31 cases of AIDS recorded. As of October 1988 this figure has risen to 1,862. In addition to those who have AIDS, some 10,000 people have been diagnosed as HIV antibody positive. The real figure is likely to be much higher. Some estimate that five times as many people living in Great Britain are already infected with HIV. Although not all of these may go on to develop AIDS or HIV-related illnesses, they could transmit the virus to others who might.

It is difficult to know whether this rapid rate of infection will continue. At the present rate, it is estimated that there will be between 10,000 and 30,000 cases of AIDS diagnosed in the United Kingdom by 1992. Whether this happens or not will depend on efforts made, both at governmental and individual levels, to prevent the transmission of HIV. In the United States the two cities with the largest numbers of AIDS cases – New York and San Francisco – appear to have levelled off in their rate of increase among gay men. However, other cities and towns, and other social groups, which have not been made as 'AIDS-aware' are still experiencing a rapid rate of increase in AIDS cases.

So what has all this got to do with women? I ask this question because until recently AIDS tended to be seen as an issue primarily affecting gay men. The media played a significant role in constructing this view, frequently referring to AIDS as the 'gay disease' or the 'gay plague'. One effect this had was to render many people at risk invisible, most especially women. In fact, while approximately three-quarters of those with AIDS in Europe and North America are gay or bisexual men, and while in some cities such as San Francisco this percentage is much higher, a significant number of women have also developed AIDS. Though very few women were affected at first, women now make up about 8 per cent of the total number of people with AIDS in the United States and the numbers are increasing. Evidence from Central Africa also challenges the idea that AIDS is something women (and heterosexuals) rarely get. Studies have shown that AIDS occurs about equally in African women and men.

So far, the number of women with AIDS in the UK is low. As of October 1988 there were 61 cases of AIDS in women.

(A similar picture exists in Australia where, by this date, 34 women were reported to have AIDS.) It is therefore difficult to say how many women are likely to be affected and how quickly. It may be that the epidemic curve will follow the pattern of that for women in the United States. Alternatively, there may be differences due to the different social conditions of British and American women at risk.

In considering how serious an issue AIDS is for women it is also important to recognise that AIDS has occurred at a time when the National Health Service is severely strained in caring for the sick. In the context of the Thatcher government's policy of cutting spending on health and social services, this is likely to place a greater burden on the 'community' providing care for people with AIDS. Traditionally it has been women who have been the main providers of community care: for children, for the elderly and for the sick.

How is HIV transmitted?

Much of the fear and panic surrounding AIDS is due to a lack of understanding of how HIV is transmitted from one person to another. Many people believe that it is possible to get AIDS through normal, everyday contact with an infected person. This is not the case. You cannot contract HIV simply by being near, eating with or touching a person who is infected by it. Nor will you become infected by touching objects used by someone who has the virus. No one has ever become infected through swimming in the same pool as an infected person, through sharing clothes or towels, or through drinking out of the same cup as them. HIV is very fragile and is easily killed outside the body. There is absolutely no reason to think that it can be spread through the air, or by casual social contact.

Perhaps the best evidence that the virus which can lead to AIDS is not passed on through ordinary everyday contact comes from health care workers who have been

treating AIDS patients for several years. There has not been
a single case of a doctor, nurse or hospital technician
developing AIDS as a result of working with AIDS patients,
and only a very few health care workers have contracted
the virus through accidentally sticking themselves with
needles or exposure of broken skin to infected blood. All
evidence indicates that it is perfectly safe to work, play, go
to school and live with people who have AIDS or are
antibody positive. If HIV could be contracted through
everyday contact there would by now be many reported
cases of AIDS, not only among health care workers, but
also among family and friends caring for people with AIDS.
Studies have shown that no friends or family members of
people with AIDS have developed AIDS themselves unless
they've had sexual contact with them or shared needles.

Most people contract HIV through having sex with
someone who is already infected with the virus. Vaginal or
anal intercourse is known to transmit the virus. Other ways
of having sex, such as oral sex, also may be risky if they
allow blood, semen or vaginal secretions containing the
virus to enter your body. Ways of reducing the risk of
infection by practising safer sex are described in Chapters 3
and 4.

It is wrong to think that HIV can only be spread through
sex between men. Despite the early association of AIDS
with gay men, we now know that the virus can be transmitted heterosexually, both from men to women and from
women to men. The occurrence of AIDS in similar numbers
among women and men in Central Africa is seen as
evidence of this, although at first researchers resisted a
sexual explanation. One theory was that blood-sucking
insects, such as mosquitoes, might carry the virus from
person to person. This has now been dismissed. HIV
infection occurs mainly in women and men of reproductive
age. People of all ages get bitten by insects.

Another explanation put forward was that the virus had
been transmitted through doctors using the same unsterile
needles on different people. The use of unscreened blood

donations has also been considered as a possible explanation of AIDS in Africa. Undoubtedly, both of these
practices are ways in which HIV could be transmitted.
Research suggests, however, that neither unscreened
blood donations nor the use of unsterile needles is the chief
means of transmission. The main way in which African
women and men appear to become infected with the virus
which can lead to AIDS is through sexual intercourse.

In addition to being able to transmit it to their heterosexual partners, women who are infected with HIV can
also pass it on to their children during pregnancy, either
through the placenta, or at birth, or possibly through their
breast milk. The relationship between pregnancy and AIDS
is discussed in the next chapter. The possibility of a woman
being able to transmit the virus to another woman sexually
has been little talked about or researched, though we
should note that lesbians are at low-risk for sexually transmitted diseases generally. This and some of the other
issues which AIDS raises for lesbians are discussed in
Chapter 3.

Apart from being seen initially as a gay disease, AIDS has
also been associated with promiscuity. For example, in
their book *AIDS: The Deadly Epidemic*, Graham Hancock and
Enver Carim state that HIV most definitely is transmitted
through 'the shared use of needles by drug abusers, and
promiscuous sex of any kind' – with an infected person of
course – (Hancock and Carim, Gollancz, 1986).

One of the problems with this is that people may con-
clude not just that if they only have sex with one person
they won't get AIDS but also that everyone infected with
HIV, or who has AIDS, must have been 'promiscuous'.
This is not the case. There are people who report having
had only one sexual encounter and have later gone on to
develop AIDS. Although the chances of your becoming
infected with HIV increase with repeated exposure, like
pregnancy you only need to have intercourse once to
contract the virus.

The word 'promiscuous' means different things to different people. It also means different things depending upon whether it is used about a woman or a man. As part of the sexual double standard that operates in our society, it is generally more acceptable for men to have more sex with more people at all ages than it is for women. Consequently, 'casual sex' in women is often seen as reprehensible in a way that it is not for men. This has important implications for who gets the blame for spreading AIDS. For example, it is women, as prostitutes, and not their male clients who have been singled out as important in the heterosexual transmission of HIV. (This is discussed in more detail in the following chapter.)

Hancock and Carim fail to specify what exactly *they* mean by 'promiscuous sex'. What they do say suggests that it is not so much the way you have sex that is important as the number of different people you have sex with. By implication, if you restrict your sexual activities to one person you ought to be OK.

Unfortunately, being monogamous is no protection against AIDS if your partner is infected with HIV and you engage in sexual acts that allow transmission of the virus. Also, monogamy is not a realistic choice for many people. Sexual relationships end for all sorts of reasons and, as a result, people will develop new ones. Young people do not always find the 'right person' the first time. Also, some may find it emotionally or economically difficult to limit sex to one person. A woman working as a prostitute, for example, would have to find an alternative way of financially supporting herself and, in many cases, her children.

Although 'promiscuity' does not cause AIDS, the number of partners you have may affect your chances of becoming infected with the virus which can lead to it. The more people you have sex with the more likely it is that at least one of them will be infected with HIV. This is especially true if you have sex with people whose behaviour puts them at risk of infection (for example, with people who inject drugs and share needles). Having said this, it is important to recognise that cutting down on the number of sexual partners one has will not significantly reduce the risks of infection with HIV if you don't also practise safer sex. It is not so much the number of people you have sex with that creates risk for infection with HIV, but what you do. Related to this, it would have been more accurate if from the beginning researchers had talked about certain kinds of behaviour being high-risk rather than certain groups of people. Not all IV drug users share needles. Not all gay men have high-risk sex.

Also, although it may be useful for targeting AIDS education, the concept of risk groups may lead some people who do not identify with these groups (but whose behaviour puts them at risk), to believe AIDS does not affect them. People get AIDS because of what they do, not because of who they are. For example, it is certain kinds of sexual activity between men that is high-risk, not being gay or bisexual. A lot of men have sex with other men and do not see themselves as gay or even bisexual. The danger is that, because their sense of identity differs, they may think that what they do does not put them at risk. This will have implications for the women, as well as the men, they have sex with – a situation made worse by the fact that many men do not tell their wives or girlfriends when they have sex with another man.

Another argument against labelling certain groups of people as 'at risk', is that it can lead not only to the belief that everyone outside of those groups is safe but also to the belief that everyone in such a group is likely to be infected. For instance, because over half of the women with AIDS in the United States are black the belief may arise that *every* black woman is at risk or infected.

HIV is passed on when blood from an infected person enters the body of an uninfected person. Apart from certain sexual practices which allow this to happen, the main risk is to drug users who share needles, syringes or other equipment used for mixing or injecting drugs.

In the past some people were given blood or blood

products which had been infected with HIV. Haemophiliacs, in particular, contracted the virus this way, through
treatment with the blood products factor 8 and factor 9
which help the blood to clot. Factor 8 is made from the
plasma of thousands of donors. Plasma is the fluid left
when the cells have been removed from the blood. Even if
only one or two of these donors are infected with HIV, the
chances are that the factor 8 produced from their blood will
also contain the virus. It is estimated that up to two-thirds
of haemophiliacs in the UK may be infected with HIV as a
result of receiving treatment with infected blood products.
As of October 1988, 123 haemophiliacs had developed
AIDS out of a total of 1,862. (In Australia haemophiliacs
make up only 1.2 per cent of the total number of people
with AIDS.) Fortunately, the risk of people contracting HIV
from infected blood products has now been eliminated.
Since 1985, all donated blood has been tested for HIV and
any blood found to be positive discarded. In addition,
blood products are heat treated, a simple process which
kills the virus.

With rare exceptions, haemophilia occurs only in men.
Very few women have therefore been at risk of contracting
HIV this way. However, as sexual partners of men with
haemophilia they may be at risk.

Before the HIV antibody test was developed, there was
also a small risk of contracting the virus through blood
transfusions. The widespread reporting of such cases in the
media immediately created generalised fear and panic.
Suddenly AIDS was no longer a disease of certain minority
groups, it was a public health issue. Anyone might conceivably need a blood transfusion sometime in their life, and
therefore anyone might conceivably become infected with
HIV and develop AIDS. One response to this scaremongering was a public appeal to all would-be donors from
'high-risk groups', urging them not to give blood. Meanwhile in the United States those who had the money to do
so began storing their own blood in case of an emergency.

Nowadays, through the use of the HIV antibody test,

blood donors are screened for infection with HIV and any blood found to be infected is rejected. As a result the risk of contracting HIV through blood transfusion has largely been eliminated. Unfortunately, this is not the case in some African countries, where the lack of effective screening of donors means that transmission of the virus through blood transfusions will continue.

Finally, as I have already mentioned, infants may be infected with HIV while in the womb or, possibly, at birth if the mother is infected. It is not yet known how many children who contract the virus from their mothers are likely to go on to develop AIDS, though some doctors have suggested that it may be as many as half.

It is important that people learn to recognise the real risks of contracting HIV and protect themselves against it. What is equally important is that people do not panic. AIDS is a preventable disease. Many women are not at risk and need worry very little about getting AIDS. Women who are at risk, or whose sexual partners are, do however need to take certain precautions.

Who gets AIDS?

AIDS occurs most commonly among gay or bisexual men in Europe and North America. Almost three-quarters of all people with AIDS in the United States and a slightly greater proportion in the UK and Australia fall into this category. This does not mean that AIDS is a gay disease. It is not. Anyone can get AIDS; heterosexual or homosexual, male or female, black or white.

In the United States the next major group are drug users who share needles, syringes or other equipment for mixing and injecting drugs. When drug users share needles blood from one user can be passed to another; if the first person has the virus it can be transmitted to the second. 'Pumping' – irrigating blood in and out of the syringe in order not to leave any of the drug behind – increases the risk of transmission.

In the United Kingdom and Australia only a few drug users have so far been reported as having AIDS. (Though still small, the number of people who have got AIDS as a result of transfusion with infected blood or blood products is greater. This group includes haemophiliacs.)

However, many IV drug users are already infected. In Australia estimates of the percentage of IV drug users thought to be HIV positive range from 2 per cent in Western Australia to between 7 and 10 per cent in New South Wales. In Edinburgh, Scotland, however, it is estimated that more than half of those who 'shoot' drugs are infected with HIV. Over the next few years we can therefore expect to see many more cases of AIDS among injecting drug users.

Sexual partners of injecting drug users, haemophiliacs and gay or bisexual men may be at risk if they have sex which allows the transmission of HIV. (For a detailed account of what kinds of sex are 'unsafe' see Chapters 3 and 4.)

Because HIV is found in semen, women who use artificial insemination by donor (AID) as a means of getting pregnant may also be at risk. They may become infected with HIV if semen from an infected donor is used. This also puts any potential offspring at risk.

Women who inseminate through a sperm bank are not likely to be at risk. Since 1985, clinics offering artificial insemination have routinely tested donors for antibodies to HIV. Women who plan to self-inseminate could however be at risk of infection with HIV if they use semen without first screening their donor. This and other issues concerning donor insemination are discussed in the following chapter.

It is extremely rare for women or men who do not fall into any of these categories to become infected with the virus which may lead to AIDS. Nevertheless, anyone who behaves in a manner which permits the transmission of HIV risks becoming infected.

What are the symptoms of AIDS?

Many of the symptoms of AIDS are similar to those that occur in common illnesses such as colds, bronchitis and stomach flu. However with AIDS these symptoms are usually more severe and last for a long time.

The general symptoms of AIDS may include:

- Profound fatigue, which lasts for weeks, with no obvious cause.
- Unexplained fever, shaking chills or drenching night sweats, lasting longer than several weeks.
- Unexpected weight loss – over ten pounds in less than two months.
- Swollen glands, especially in the neck or armpits.
- Thrush (*Candida*) – creamy white blotches or sores in the mouth or throat. Thrush is a common vaginal infection among women, causing an irritating white discharge.

  In men, thrush may appear as irritating white spots on the end of the penis or as a white discharge from the rectum.
- Persistent diarrhoea.
- Shortness of breath, gradually getting worse over several weeks, together with a dry, irritating cough that is not from smoking and has lasted longer than it would if it were just from a bad cold.
- New pink or purple, flat or raised blotches (usually painless) occurring anywhere on the skin, including on the mouth or eyelids. In many cases lesions can also be found internally, such as, for example, on the membranes of the lung, intestines or rectum. Initially they may look like blood blisters or bruises, but they do not pale when pressed and do not disappear. They are usually harder than the skin around them. This is a form of skin cancer known as Kaposi's sarcoma. For reasons that are not fully understood, it is not a common symptom in women with AIDS.

If you have some of these symptoms don't be alarmed, it does not mean that you must have AIDS. There can be lots of other reasons for nearly all of these symptoms. For instance, swollen glands can be a sign of glandular fever and tiredness; and fever and weight loss are much more likely to be symptoms of stress, exhaustion or of a cold coming on. If, however, you do have some of the above symptoms and think there is a possibility that you might have been infected with HIV, you should see a doctor, preferably one who is familiar with AIDS. A clinic which specialises in genito-urinary infections may be able to provide this. You can get the address of your nearest clinic by looking in the phone book under VD (venereal disease) or STD (sexually transmitted disease). You could also contact a local AIDS organisation for advice (see page 184 for a list of AIDS organisations).

Can AIDS be treated?

There is currently no treatment that will destroy HIV or restore the immune system. Research on antiviral drugs is being carried out in the United States and other countries in an attempt to provide a cure. Antiviral drugs are substances which interfere with the growth and reproduction of viruses. One problem with such drugs has been that they often do not discriminate between infected cells and healthy cells. In order to be effective an antiviral drug would need to attack only infected cells, leaving healthy cells undamaged. Another problem is that HIV is capable of infecting cells in the brain and other parts of the central nervous system. If an antiviral drug is not capable of passing through into the brain or cerebrospinal fluid, and most are not, these infected cells may continue to produce more and more viruses.

Even if an antiviral drug capable of reaching the brain and cerebrospinal fluid were developed, there would still be problems. HIV incorporates itself into the genetic code of the cells it infects. As there is no way of disentangling the virus from the genetic code of the host cells, the only means of getting rid of HIV is to kill all of the cells it has infected. This becomes very difficult once the virus has entered the brain, as it would mean killing off vital brain cells.

Some of the antiviral drugs which are being researched have prompted a temporary remission in people with AIDS. Preliminary studies of the drug Ribavarin, for example, have shown that it can slow down production of HIV. Further research is under way to assess its possible usefulness in the treatment of AIDS. Tests on other antiviral agents, such as Suramin, HPA–23 and Ansamycin, have also demonstrated a reduction in the amount of virus present. Unfortunately, although certain antiviral drugs may help to slow down the progress of the disease, none of the drugs tested so far looks like providing a miracle cure for AIDS. More likely, a successful cure will come from a combination of various drugs and therapies.

In addition to the antiviral drugs already being tested, research is also being carried out on drugs which influence the immune system. Some of these are immune-boosting drugs, such as Interferon. Others, like Cyclosporin, act by suppressing the immune system. This latter approach to treatment stems from the theory that HIV works by tricking the immune system into destroying itself. By slowing down the immune system some researchers believe one might also slow down or stop this process of immune self-destruction. The possibility that bone marrow transplantation (in conjunction with treatment with antiviral drugs) may restore immune functioning in some people with AIDS is also under investigation.

HIV needs an enzyme called *reverse transcriptase* in order to multiply. A drug that stops this enzyme from working should stop the virus reproducing itself. AZT is thought to work in this way. Made by Burroughs Wellcome, AZT has been tested mainly on AIDS patients who have pneumonia. AZT is not a cure for AIDS. Although it stops the virus from multiplying, it does not destroy it. It may also induce serious side-effects, such as severe anaemia. It is also not clear what the long-term consequences of taking AZT will be. It does, however, appear to have been successful in prolonging the lives of some AIDS patients.

There is not yet a cure for AIDS, but the infections and cancers associated with AIDS can be treated with varying degrees of success. These treatments include antibiotics, chemotherapy, radiation therapy and experimental techniques. Unfortunately, many of these treatments have side-effects. Also, because there is no way of correcting the underlying immune deficiency, when a person is treated for and cured of an infection it does not mean they won't become ill again. They still have AIDS and will be susceptible to further opportunistic infections or cancers.

One of the most common illnesses found in people with AIDS is pneumocystic carinii pneumonia (PCP). If caught early pneumocystis can be effectively treated with antibiotics. The standard treatment for PCP is with Septra or Pentamidine. These drugs often produce serious side-effects which include rashes, fatigue and nausea. Some people respond well to treatment while others may feel ill from the drugs and take longer to recover. In some cases doctors are trying to prevent recurrence of PCP by keeping people with AIDS on prolonged courses of antibiotics. Doctors are also experimenting with using aerosol pentamidine which can be inhaled into the lungs and, whilst effective in preventing PCP, appears to have few side-effects.

Another common symptom of AIDS, especially in men, is Kaposi's sarcoma. Treatment for this involves both radiation therapy and chemotherapy. Whilst in some cases this is effective, there may be side-effects such as hair loss, vomiting and nausea. A further problem with one of the drugs used to treat Kaposi's sarcoma, Vinblastine, is that it suppresses the immune system. This can mean that although the cancer may be treated, the body's immunity to infection is lowered even further, allowing other life-threatening illnesses such as pneumocystis to take hold.

Despite the fact that people with AIDS are often successfully treated for the infections and cancers associated with AIDS and may lead active lives for long periods of time, the harsh reality is that no one has yet been known to recover from AIDS. Most people die within two to three years of being diagnosed. Faced with this, a number of people with AIDS or other HIV-related illness combine conventional medical treatment with a holistic approach. The holistic approach to health aims to treat the 'whole person' – physically, emotionally, spiritually and mentally – by getting the body to use its natural forces to heal itself. Holistic treatment of AIDS focuses on the underlying cause of the illness, the destruction of the body's natural defence systems, and seeks to restore the immune system through alternative therapies. These include getting enough rest, taking regular exercise; maintaining a healthy diet by cutting out things like sugar, caffeine and alcohol; acupuncture; vitamin therapy; stress reduction and learning to 'think positive'.

Those people with AIDS who follow holistic treatments experience the same sad outcome as those undergoing traditional treatment, a gradual weakening of the body and eventually death. However, some people feel that holistic therapies allow them to maintain their health and a high quality of life for a longer period than would be the case if they were only having chemotherapy or other medical treatments. They may feel more in control of their lives and their health. Because they encourage people's efforts to help themselves, such regimes may also give a person greater hope.

Another goal in the treatment of AIDS is the development of a vaccine that would induce lasting immunity to HIV and thus prevent AIDS. This probably won't be produced until the 1990s at the earliest. Although the development of such a vaccine is proceeding, it faces major obstacles. When a vaccine is injected into the bloodstream a small amount of a bacteria or virus (in this case HIV) is released, causing the body to produce antibodies. These antibodies remain in the blood ready to stop any future infection occurring. They do this by locking into the outer coat of infectious organisms, thereby rendering them harmless. One of the characteristics of HIV is that it is constantly mutating and producing different strains with different outer coatings. If the antibodies being produced no longer fit the lock on the outer coat of the virus they will be unable to do their job. Even if a vaccine is produced, therefore, it may still not offer the ultimate solution. The fact that the virus keeps changing could mean that the vaccine would quickly become ineffective against new strains of HIV. A further problem in finding a vaccine, and a cure, is that the antibodies to HIV don't actually kill the virus. Normally, antibodies destroy viruses and it is one of the unusual features of HIV, and something that researchers cannot at present explain, that the antibodies appear ineffective.

Research is continuing to try to produce a vaccine. However, even if a vaccine were produced tomorrow, it would take years of development and testing before it would become widely available. Prevention through education and behaviour change may be the only effective defence against AIDS for some time to come.

2 AIDS in women

Women make up approximately 8 per cent of the total number of AIDS cases in the United States. Because this is a relatively small proportion, AIDS in women often tends to get overlooked. This is also true of Australia and the UK where, at present, the number of women with AIDS is low. The fact that in Africa several thousand women have AIDS is not the only reason why this silence needs to be challenged. In addition to those who have already developed AIDS, many more women are infected with the virus which causes it or are concerned and worried that they might contract it. Women need to know as much as possible about AIDS and what they can do to protect themselves.

Very little research has been done on the pattern of infection in women. One ongoing study which has looked at this is the San Francisco-based community study known as project AWARE (Association for Women's AIDS Research and Education). The aim of this study is to find out which women are particularly at risk for HIV infection as a result of heterosexual contact, by testing for antibodies to the virus. Over 550 women have taken part in the study so far. They have either had a heterosexual relationship with a man at risk for AIDS in the last three years or have had multiple sexual relationships with men. For the purposes of this study this was defined as five or more sexual partners in the previous three years. Women have not been recruited for the study directly. Instead, women who feel they may be at risk are encouraged to call in and discuss their own risk situation and the project. Those who agree to take part are interviewed about sexual and lifestyle practices that are associated with AIDS – such as sharing needles to inject drugs – and are given the antibody test. Preliminary reports show 5 per cent to be antibody positive. Although this is too small a number to say anything very definite it is worth noting that, compared to women who had a negative test result, the 'postive' group were more likely to have had bisexual or injecting, drug-using sexual partners, or partners with AIDS. They were also more likely to have injected drugs themselves.

Up to the end of October 1988 there were 61 cases of women with AIDS in the UK, including ten girls. In Australia the figure for women with AIDS is 34 (August 1988). In the United States over 6,000 women have so far been reported to have the disease. Some doctors think the real figure may be higher. One reason for possible under-reporting is that many doctors don't expect women to develop AIDS. There is also the possibility that because AIDS was largely defined in terms of symptoms first seen in gay men, the opportunistic infections that may be part of the spectrum of AIDS-related diseases in women go unrecognised.

The largest group of women with AIDS in the United States are women who inject drugs, just over half of the total cases among women. Of the rest, 29 per cent are women who have had sexual contact with men with AIDS or who are at risk for AIDS; 11 per cent are women who have received transfusions with infected blood. The remaining 8 per cent are women for whom no specific risk was identified. This includes women with incomplete medical histories. Also, some women who have developed AIDS may not wish to admit being at risk. They may be too afraid or embarrassed to say that they inject drugs, for instance, or have a boyfriend or husband who is bisexual.

Over half of the women with AIDS in the United States are in New York City or New Jersey, about 10 per cent are in Miami, and the rest are scattered across the country. The vast majority are young women between twenty and forty years old. AIDS also affects a lot more black and Hispanic women. For men with AIDS a greater percentage are white (61 per cent) than are black (24 per cent) or Hispanic (14 per cent). Of the women who have so far been diagnosed with AIDS 51 per cent are black, 20 per cent latina and 28 per cent white (July 1988). A small number are Asian, Native American, or from other backgrounds.

That 73 per cent of women with AIDS in the United States are black or latina is clearly disproportionate to the percentage of the population which they represent. According to health officials, this reflects the more widespread use of injectable drugs among black and Hispanic women. It may also be because the social conditions of many black and latina women's lives, poverty and poor access to health education and care included, put them at greater risk. In the context of the discrimination which black and latina women already face, it is important that this is understood. All too often researchers ignore the wider social conditions, including poverty, racism and sexism, which are at the roots of the spread of AIDS in the black and Hispanic community.

To summarise, women are at risk of acquiring the virus which can lead to AIDS if they:

- Inject drugs and share their 'works'.
- Have unprotected sexual intercourse with, or are artificially inseminated by, a man who is infected with HIV.
- Receive a blood transfusion with blood infected with HIV. (In the UK and the United States the risk of infection has now been largely eliminated.)

Injecting drug users

Women who inject drugs are at risk for AIDS (and other diseases) if they share needles, syringes or other equipment used for mixing and injecting drugs. Many drug users who inject drugs do share needles. Unfortunately, if you inject yourself using an unsterilised needle which has previously been used by someone infected with HIV you could become infected yourself. (Sharing ear-piercing equipment and tattooing, electrolysis and acupuncture needles may carry some degree of risk. It is important to check that practitioners sterilise equipment that is re-used.)

It is not only intravenous (IV) drug use which carries this risk. Injecting yourself anywhere could lead to the virus being passed on (this includes skin-popping). Irrigating blood in and out of the syringe in order not to leave behind any of the drug it contains is likely to increase the chances of this happening.

In the United States women who inject drugs and share their 'works' run the greatest risk of developing AIDS. By October 1988, 6,260 women in the United States had AIDS. Half of these were women IV drug users. So far there have been very few cases of AIDS among injecting drug users in the UK. Only 11 women are reported to have developed AIDS as a result of sharing equipment to inject drugs (by October 1988). Over the next few years, however, it is likely that we will see a growing number of women who inject drugs develop AIDS or HIV-related illness. The DHSS estimate that in England 10 per cent, on average, of those who inject drugs are already infected with HIV (October 1988). In some parts of the UK this figure may be even higher. In Edinburgh, for example, studies suggest that more than half of the city's injecting users may be infected. This reflects the difficulties which those injecting drugs have had, in the past, in obtaining sterile needles and syringes, causing many to risk infection with HIV by sharing their works – an unfortunate outcome of police attempts to regulate drug use by limiting the availability of hypodermic needles. Similarly in New York, where it is a crime to buy or carry a needle without a doctor's prescription, many IV drug users go to 'shooting galleries', where needles and syringes may be hired and are frequently shared by large numbers of users.

Many women who inject drugs are doubly at risk of getting AIDS. Drug use puts women directly at risk where they themselves inject drugs and share dirty and possibly infected works. As sexual partners of men who inject drugs women are also at risk. As I have already mentioned, the virus can be transmitted from a man to a woman during vaginal or anal intercourse. Women who make love with men who inject drugs should therefore practise 'safer sex'. (A full discussion of what is safe and what is risky sex is provided in Chapter 4.) Otherwise, however much care *they* take not to share their works, they could still become infected through sex.

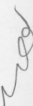

Some women who inject drugs, especially if they are poor and homeless, may have little to trade besides sex to get money for drugs. They may be at risk of HIV infection if they use prostitution as a means of financing their drug habit and don't take precautions.

Drug users who are antibody positive have sometimes been denied surgical operations, dental treatment and other forms of medical care, including treatment for their drug problems. Such unsympathetic treatment stems in part from the unfounded fears which some health workers have that they may contract HIV from patients who are infected with the virus. It may also be related to the assumption that drug users get what they deserve because they use drugs. Gay men have also been subjected to similar kinds of injustice. In their case, however, it is homophobic beliefs that homosexuality is abnormal, sick or morally wrong that have led some to make the frighteningly insensitive claim that AIDS is no more than what they deserve.

Whilst the virus must be present in the body for AIDS to occur, infection with HIV does not always lead to the development of AIDS or HIV-related illness. It is possible that other as yet unknown factors, which also affect the immune system, may play a part in determining who goes on to develop AIDS once they have been infected with HIV, and who does not. Drug users use substances which suppress the immune system. Some researchers believe that this may increase the chances of those infected with

HIV progressing to AIDS. Poor nutrition has also been suggested as a possible co-factor. Where there is an association between drug taking and poverty or drug taking and eating disorders – as often seems to be the case in women – there may therefore be a further risk.

One way of avoiding these risks is to stop using drugs. For many women this will be very hard to do, but some do manage to stop with the help and support of others. If you are thinking about coming off drugs there are a number of organisations which you could contact to help you (see page 187).

A very effective way of reducing the risks of contracting HIV and possibly developing AIDS if you don't feel able to give up drugs is not to inject. If you stop injecting drugs you are completely safe from becoming infected with HIV through taking drugs. You cannot get HIV from sniffing, snorting, smoking or swallowing drugs. There are other reasons for stopping injecting besides AIDS. Hepatitis, blood poisoning, endocarditis (an infection of the heart), and nerve damage are some of the other health problems associated with injecting drugs.

If coming off or changing the way you use drugs are choices you don't feel able to make then you should stop sharing. Don't rent works as they may have been used by lots of people. Don't use rebagged needles. Buy a new needle and don't let anyone else use it. If you do use someone else's works, or they use yours, clean them throughly before injecting. Don't believe they've been cleaned unless you've cleaned them yourself. Since people may transmit the virus without showing any symptoms, sharing needles with someone who appears healthy is not a safeguard.

This applies whether you inject drugs regularly or only occasionally, and is something everyone can do. Don't make the mistake of one woman I spoke to who, although she injected drugs and shared needles, didn't consider herself at risk of infection because, as she put it, 'I'm not a *user*, I only shoot drugs now and again.'

Similarly, a woman may not consider herself to be sharing if she only shares a set of works with her partner. Unfortunately this will be no protection if he is already infected, or is at risk of infection through *his* sharing with other IV drug users.

It may help to label or mark your works so that both you and other people know which are yours. Care should also be taken not to mix your gear up in a spoon or mixing bowl used by other people. When you have used a needle and syringe, bend back the needle and dispose of it safely. Do not leave used needles lying around where people can accidentally stab themselves or where others might find and use them.

Even with the knowledge of the risk of becoming infected with HIV, circumstances can arise where sharing is likely. You may be new to drugs and haven't yet got your own works. You may be frightened that if you do you'll become addicted. You may not have your works with you. You may fear others finding out about your drug habit, or being arrested, if you carry your works. If you are going to share, cleaning the works *before* you use them will reduce the risk of infection. Clean used or borrowed works by soaking the needle, syringe and cooker in rubbing alcohol (at least 40 per cent alcohol) or in a mixture of household bleach and water (one part bleach to ten parts water) for at least ten minutes. (Draw the alcohol or bleach through the needle and squirt it out several times before soaking.) Then rinse the works in running tap water. You must get rid of all the bleach solution or alcohol from the works before you use them. Never inject alcohol or bleach into the body.

It is essential that women who inject drugs have access to information and advice about AIDS. This is especially true of girls who, if they are to become aware of the risks associated with experimenting with injectable drugs, must be given information about AIDS and how it is spread. Apart from public education campaigns, which should include guidelines for both safer sex and safer drug use, counselling and advisory services are needed. These should provide advice to women about how to reduce the risk of HIV infection to themselves and, if they are already infected, to others. This will include being told that if they are infected there is a high chance they may pass the virus on to any future children they may have. Also, that pregnancy may possibly increase their own chances of developing AIDS. A woman who injects drugs, *or whose sexual partner injects drugs*, will need counselling about these issues as well as advice about birth control. Some women who have stopped taking drugs may also be anxious to know whether or not they became infected with HIV whilst they were injecting drugs and will need counselling about whether or not they should take the antibody test.

Half the difficulty with AIDS prevention is getting the message across. This will not be easy with drug users who may already be at risk of early death through injecting drugs, and when any future danger of AIDS seems less important than the day-to-day problems of poverty and drug use. As one woman said, 'How can I worry about something that will kill me in five years when I don't know if I'll be alive in the morning.'

In order to inform IV drug users about AIDS a large network must be used, including other drug users and ex-users, schools and jails. The advice should be clear, easy to understand and *relevant*. For many IV drug users, some of the recommendations are a million miles from the kind of lives they lead. It's not surprising many women drug users distrust those offering help and advice, especially if the information they are given is aimed at changing their behaviour not risk-reduction. Some women may also be frightened that if they seek help or information about their drug habits their children will be taken into care. The problem is even worse for black women for whom the experience of racism is likely to discourage seeking help for drug-related problems.

Acknowledging the difficulties of targeting AIDS information at IV drug users, some believe that preventing the sharing of equipment may be the quickest and most effective means of limiting the transmission of HIV among injecting drug users. In parts of the UK needle exchange schemes have been set up as an attempt to reduce the sharing of infected equipment. IV drug users are given a new sterile injection kit free of charge when they hand in their old needles, as well as advice on safer sex or drug use. Similar schemes exist in parts of Australia. In Australian Capital Territory and Western Australia, for example, there are also needle exchange buses which tour the area.

Others have argued against the development of such schemes on the grounds that they will encourage and increase drug use. In the United States, for example, the approach the Reagan administration has taken is to recommend abstinence. Unfortunately, this will not work. It is unrealistic, and naive, to simply tell people 'say no to drugs' and expect them to be able to do so. Even those who advocate needle exchange schemes to try to reduce sharing recognise that getting people to change their drug habits is not that simple. For example, another way one might reduce the sharing of equipment, at least among some users, would be to prescribe the non-injectable drug methadone as a substitute for heroin. However, it is important to understand that this involves both giving up dependency on a particular drug *and* the habit of injecting. Habits, as we all know, are hard to break.

There needs to be a multi-faceted approach towards reducing the rate of HIV infection among IV drug users. Alongside schemes to try to reduce needle sharing, there need to be education programmes targeted specifically at drug users as well as more drug treatment centres to help people either come off or change the way they use drugs.

Sexual transmission

Although it has played a limited role in the spread of AIDS in Europe and the United States to date, heterosexual transmission of HIV is possible.

In Australia, in 1985, reports that four women had been infected with HIV as a result of being artificially insemi-nated with semen from an infected donor provided con-vincing evidence of male to female transmission. Since then, studies in the United States and Europe have shown that sexual transmission has occurred from men, par-ticularly injecting drug users, to their female partners.

Evidence of sexual transmission of the virus from women to men is more sketchy. We know that HIV is present in the vaginal and cervical fluids of infected women, and that sexual transmission of the virus from women to men can occur. In one case a woman who had received a kidney transplant from an HIV-infected kidney donor passed the virus on to her husband who was at no other apparent risk of infection other than sexual intercourse with his wife. Several cases have also been reported where men appear to have developed AIDS through sexual contact with women who injected drugs. It is not clear whether these men contracted HIV, which led to their developing AIDS, from blood associated with sex or from vaginal secretions.

Many researchers believe that it is easier for a man to transmit the virus to a woman during intercourse than it is for a woman to pass it on to a man. Such claims are largely based on the number of reported cases, rather than on any direct evidence comparing rates of infection among the sexual partners of HIV-infected women with those of HIV-infected men. In the United States, for example, sex with a woman infected with HIV has been strongly implicated as the source of AIDS in 473 men (October 1988). This number represents approximately 0.7 per cent of all AIDS cases among men in the United States. A further 892 men listed by the CDC under the category 'heterosexual cases' are presumed to have acquired AIDS through hetero-sexual transmission. These are men without other identi-fied risks, who were born in countries where AIDS is thought to be spread mainly by heterosexual intercourse (i.e., Haiti and countries in Central Africa). By contrast, the number of women thought to have developed AIDS through sexual contact with a man was 1,558, approximately 25 per cent of the total number of women with AIDS. (A further 282 women were included under the category 'heterosexual cases'. These were immigrants from countries in which heterosexual transmission is believed to play a major role.) What this indicated is that while heterosexual contact has to date been relatively unimportant in the spread of AIDS among men, in women it is a significant risk factor. Of the 2,031 total reported people with AIDS in the United States whose only risk factor is heterosexual contact with a person at risk for AIDS, over 75 per cent are women (October 1988).

These statistics are probably a reflection of the fact that, at present, more men are infected than women. But research also suggests that vaginal and cervical secretions may be less effective transmitters of HIV than either semen or blood which contain higher concentrations of the virus. Anatomically too, there is possibly more opportunity for the virus to gain entry to the bloodstream of a woman than a man during intercourse. Providing she is not menstruating, it would seem that the virus is less likely to be sexually transmitted from a woman to a man than vice versa. (This is one reason why sex between women is likely to be safer than heterosexual intercourse.)

The actual mechanism by which the virus gets into a woman's bloodstream, and the relative efficiency for male-female and female-male transmission, is not known. The virus might enter the bloodstream through ulcerations or erosions of the cervix or through the vaginal walls which become swollen with blood during sexual arousal. Cuts or sores on a woman's genital area may also allow infected semen to reach the bloodstream. For this reason the virus may be acquired more easily by women who have venereal infections, such as herpes or gonorrhoea. There may be other factors which may increase a woman's risk of infection. Birth control pills, for example, significantly increase the risk of a woman getting certain sexually transmitted diseases, such as gonorrhoea. Research needs to be done to examine whether, in addition to its other health risks, taking the pill puts women at greater risk of contracting HIV.

The virus may also be transmitted more easily by women with infections which cause a discharge containing virus-infected cells. Because the virus is found in blood, HIV may also be present in the vagina in greater quantities during a woman's period. As with male-female transmission, the virus may be passed more easily from a woman to a man during intercourse if there are cuts or abrasions on the penis or the urethra which would allow the virus more direct access to the bloodstream.

Apart from not knowing how the virus actually gets into a woman's bloodstream during sex, there are also many unanswered questions about the relative risk that different sexual activities may carry. Some practices are thought to transmit the virus more readily than others. Anal inter-course often causes tearing of tissue and, some experts believe, may allow more of the virus in semen to enter the bloodstream directly. But vaginal intercourse is clearly the cause of infection in many women.

Whether the virus can be transmitted orally, either by oral-genital or oral-anal contact, is not clear. (There is no evidence to suggest oral transmission through kissing.) One of the difficulties in trying to study this is that people who have oral sex very often also engage in other kinds of sex which would allow transmission of the virus such as, for instance, vaginal intercourse.

The percentage of women in the United States who have been diagnosed with AIDS as a result of heterosexual contact has risen sharply from 18 per cent of all female cases in 1986 to 29 per cent in 1988. In the UK, 24 out of the 61 cases of AIDS in women so far reported have been attri-buted to heterosexual contact (October 1988). A similar pattern to that in the United States may emerge as more women who have been infected with HIV develop AIDS.

The women at risk are sexual partners of gay or bisexual men who have high-risk sex, IV drug users who share their works, recipients of infected blood or blood products (which includes men with haemophilia) and men who have had high-risk sex in countries where HIV seems to be primarily transmitted by heterosexual intercourse. The other group who are potentially at risk are women who have sex with many different men, particularly if they don't know much about them and engage in 'unsafe' sex.

Sexual partners of men at risk

Women who are sexual partners of men with AIDS, or men who are at risk of acquiring the syndrome, are themselves at risk. Studies both in the United States and the UK suggest that about 10 per cent of women with male partners with haemophilia, who have been infected with HIV through receiving treatment with infected blood products, are likely to be antibody positive themselves. To further reduce the risk of infection care should be taken to make love in ways that are safe.

Women can also become infected with HIV through sexual contact with men who inject drugs and share their works. Of the women in the United States who have got AIDS through sex with men, the majority had partners who were injecting drug users. The next largest group were female partners of bisexual men.

For reasons that are not entirely clear, female partners of men who are IV drug users appear to have a higher rate of infection (studies suggest about 40 per cent) than female partners of haemophiliac men, men infected through blood transfusions or bisexual men. It is difficult to know what these findings mean. One possible explanation is that inadequate health care or poor living conditions may affect susceptibility to infection and may account for higher rates of infection in partners of IV drug users. Until the reasons for these differences are better understood, we should be careful not to generalise about the IV drug-using population as a whole. This is particularly important given the discrimination which already exists towards IV drug users.

The potential for transmission of HIV from men to their female sexual partners is one of the few areas where research related to women and AIDS is ongoing. At the University of California, Berkeley, Nancy Padian is conducting a study of women partners of men infected with HIV or who have AIDS. A high proportion of the men in the study are bisexual. Of the 100 or so women who have so far taken part, approximately 20 per cent have been infected by their partners, since no other risk factors have been identified. (It is not known why some women with the same history of exposure to the virus become infected and others do not.) A similar study involving the partners of bisexual men is being carried out at the Middlesex Hospital, London.

Because they represent a possible route of infection from gay men to the wider heterosexual community, bisexual men have had a great deal of hostility directed at them. What we should also remember, of course, is that a considerable number of men who consider themselves heterosexual have sex with men from time to time.

Criticisms of bisexuality have not just come from the heterosexual world. Some lesbians are concerned that bisexual women may introduce AIDS into the lesbian community. This, and some of the other issues which AIDS raises for lesbians, are discussed in more detail in the following chapter.

It seems that, *at present*, there is a greater risk of a woman getting AIDS if she has a steady sexual relationship with one man who is infected with HIV than if she has sex with many different partners. (This reflects the current low level of HIV infection among heterosexual men, at least in Europe and the United States.) For example, in one case where a 71-year-old woman developed AIDS, her only apparent risk factor was infrequent sexual intercourse with her husband, a 74-year-old haemophiliac who had received factor 8 concentrate. This woman had sex only with her husband, to whom she had been married for more than fifty years. Apart from demonstrating that AIDS can occur in the elderly as well as in young people, what this shows is that even if you have sex only occasionally, or with just one person, it is still possible to get AIDS if your partner is infected with HIV.

While repeated sexual contact with one infected partner increases the likelihood of your becoming infected, it is also the case that the more people you have sex with the more likely it is that at least one of them will be infected with the virus. For this reason women who have sex with many different men, whether for payment or not, are also at greater risk of *exposure* to HIV. However, having more than one sexual partner does not automatically increase a woman's risk of *infection* if she is practising safer sex. Prostitutes do not appear to have a higher risk of infection than other women if they are using safe sex practices in their work and do not inject drugs and share their works.

Another kind of risk assessment therefore is what kind of sexual practices do you engage in? You are most at risk of contracting HIV if you have vaginal or anal intercourse, especially if your male partner does not use a condom.

In the San Francisco-based AWARE study, over half of the women said that they had had anal intercourse with one or more men. Whilst this included women who worked in the sex industry and women who did not, the former were much more likely to have used a condom. In general, women working as prostitutes reported more use of barrier protection methods for all types of sexual behaviour.

These findings, though preliminary, provide a useful introduction to the more general issue of prostitution and AIDS.

Prostitutes

Although there were, in 1988, over 6,000 women in the United States with AIDS and several thousand reported in

Africa, very little research has been done on who, among
women, is likely to get AIDS and how. Some women at risk
have been identified, such as women who share equipment
for injecting drugs, but others such as prostitutes are being
named regardless of the fact that so far there is little direct
evidence that they are a 'risk group'. Even if they were it
would be wrong to single out prostitutes as a distinct
group. It is certain kinds of sexual contact which transmit
the virus, not the exchange of money for carrying them out.

There have been a number of studies that have looked at
the rate of infection among prostitutes. Only one out of
over 100 prostitutes tested at a London hospital had antibodies to HIV, and she had shared equipment for injecting
drugs. In West Germany, only 1 per cent of nearly 2,000
registered prostitutes who were tested were antibody positive and almost all of these used IV drugs. In the United
States, the rates of infection reported on the East Coast
have been relatively high. One New Jersey study found 32
out of 56 prostitutes who were tested to be sero-positive. A
problem with this and a number of other studies is that
since the women taking part were recruited at methadone
maintenance clinics they were neither representative of
prostitutes in the United States as a whole nor even of New
Jersey. The prostitutes who were infected were IV drug
users.

The figures reported on the West Coast have been much
lower. In San Francisco, only 5 per cent of the prostitutes
taking part in the AWARE study were antibody positive.
Apart from including a wider cross-section of the prostitute
population than most studies, this study also tested women
with 'multiple sexual partners' who were not prostitutes.
The proportion of women found to be positive was the
same: 5 per cent. There was a difference, however, between
the two groups of women in terms of past drug use. All of
the prostitutes who tested positive had a history of IV drug
use, while some non-prostitutes who were infected did not.

In Africa the situation appears to be rather different.
Studies of prostitutes in several countries in Central Africa

report relatively high rates of infection. One possible explanation for this difference is the use of condoms. In Europe
and the United States prostitutes routinely use condoms
with customers. In parts of Central Africa condoms are not
as easily available, partly because of their cost and partly
because of cultural reasons. An alternative explanation for
the different pattern of infection in Africa is the higher
prevalence of untreated sexually transmitted diseases that
seem to facilitate transmission of HIV.

Studies such as these suggest that in the West unless a
prostitute injects drugs she is unlikely to be infected with
HIV. Although only a minority of prostitutes are IV drug
users, some women who are 'on the game' use prostitution
as a way of getting drugs or money to pay for drugs. In New
York, for instance, injecting drugs is reported to be most
common among the groups of prostitutes known as 'street-
walkers'. It is estimated that in the United States about 10 to
20 per cent of prostitution involves street prostitutes. These
are women who pick up their clients on the street rather
than through, say, an escort agency. As a high proportion
(some estimate as many as half) of the city's injecting drug
users are believed to be infected with the virus, this may
explain why some street prostitutes in New York, and cities
like it, are reported to be at risk.

A large number of street prostitutes are working-class
and black women. While this is partly related to poverty, it
is also due to the racism which prevents black prostitutes
from working indoors in brothels and casinos, or for escort
agencies. It is street prostitutes who, because they are more
'visible', have particularly suffered from increased violence
and harassment and, consequently, loss of earnings which
has been one result of blaming prostitutes for spreading
AIDS.

In many ways, it is ironic that prostitutes have been
scapegoated for AIDS. Contrary to popular belief, prostitutes are often among the best informed as to how to
protect themselves and others from sexually transmitted
diseases, including AIDS. After all, it makes good business

and health sense for them to know. Also, while it is a common assumption that prostitutes spend most of their time engaging in high-risk sex with their customers, few studies exist of what men specifically pay prostitutes to do for them.

Claims that prostitutes are spreading AIDS need to be understood in relation to beliefs about both prosititution and AIDS. To be a prostitute is to belong to a normally despised category of women which (like homosexuality) has long been linked with disease and contagion. The image of a woman who sells sex for money is often that of someone who is unclean and spreads infection and is immoral. During the hunt for the Yorkshire Ripper, Peter Sutcliffe, for example, both the police and the press sought to make a distinction between the killing of 'innocent' women and the killing of prostitutes.

AIDS has often been talked about, especially by certain sections of the mass media, in a way that is equally judgmental. The assumption that AIDS is the result of bad behaviour pervades the perception of it as a disease trans- mitted by, presumably guilty, 'carriers' such as homosex- uals, drug users and prostitutes, to 'innocent victims', such as haemophiliacs, receivers of blood transfusions and infants. In this view it is the actions of certain groups of people that cause AIDS, not a virus.

Initially, it was gay men who were blamed for AIDS. This ensured that gay men who got AIDS, of which there have been a great many, received little public sympathy. Not only was it seen as their own fault that they had become ill but also, and of far more interest to the heterosexual majority, it was perceived as their fault that those who were not gay developed AIDS. 'Homosexuals' – and this included lesbians – were judged to be guilty of spreading the disease to others.

With the growing recognition that AIDS is not a 'gay disease' and can be transmitted heterosexually, a new scapegoat became necessary. Women prostitutes appar- ently fitted the bill nicely.

Although female prostitutes have been blamed for the spread of AIDS, few if any cases of AIDS in men can be unequivocally linked to them. Arguably, if infected prostitutes were transmitting the virus to their customers we ought by now to see many thousands of heterosexual men infected. In the United States, men whose only known risk is that they say they have had sex with a prostitute are listed by the Centers for Disease Control in Atlanta, Georgia, as at 'no identified risk'. As of October 1988 only 3 per cent of all the men in the United States who had AIDS fell into this category, a total of 1,920. That about a third of these say they have a history of visiting prostitutes is difficult to interpret. A lot of men who have got AIDS may not wish to admit to being at risk in other ways. For instance, given that it is generally seen as both more understandable and more acceptable for a man to pay a woman to have sex with him than it is for a man to desire another man, some men may claim to have got the virus from a prostitute because it is much less difficult than saying that they are bisexual or gay. This may be particularly true of soldiers, who according to some studies, claim they have become infected as a result of sexual contact with a prositute. In the United States military, both homosexuality and IV drug use are grounds for discharge.

Another possible explanation is that men who visit prostitutes could be infecting each other. Very few men in the United States are known to have become infected through sexual contact with a woman. Semen, however, has been shown to be a very effective means of transmitting the HIV virus. It could be that infected semen remaining in the vagina from one customer could later infect another customer.

The possibility that a prostitute might contract HIV from a customer, though rarely discussed, is something most prostitutes are aware of. Leading AIDS experts advise women against sexual contact with men who may be at risk. Those women who, like prostitutes, are not always in a position to be able to follow this advice should practise safe sex to reduce their risk of infection. The problem with this is that a man may take the view that if he has paid for sex he's entitled to have the kind of sex he wants. Many men, for instance, don't like using condoms and may refuse to wear one. Some may even offer extra money to have sex without a condom. While most prostitutes do use condoms, some women may agree to do this, even though it puts them at risk, because they are desperate for the money. This is likely to be especially true of women for whom prostitution is the only way they can get enough money to pay for heroin or other drugs. What is also needed, therefore, is AIDS education aimed at men who visit prostitutes to convince them of the need to use condoms so they will no longer argue against using them.

Those who regard prostitutes as responsible for the spread of AIDS tend to ignore men's involvement in prostitution. This has happened before. In the mid nineteenth century concerns about the incidence of venereal disease among British soldiers led to the passing of the Contagious Diseases Acts. Under the terms of these Acts it was women suspected of being prostitutes, and not soldiers, who were required to register and have regular medical examinations. The Acts were vigorously opposed by feminists like Josephine Butler as clearly unfair to women. They upheld a sexual double standard, which still exists today, by seeking to regulate women while ignoring men's role in the spread of venereal disease.

In much the same way it is prostitutes and not their male clients who are now being blamed for the spread of AIDS. Again the concern is that this may lead to new forms of social control of women. With the introduction of blood testing for antibodies to HIV, the possibility of introducing registration and compulsory testing of prostitutes obviously exists. Similarly, the government might allow the use of quarantine to isolate women with HIV or AIDS whom, it might be feared, might continue to work as prostitutes.

This is not as far-fetched as it might seem. Some members of parliament, concerned about AIDS, have called for brothels to be made legal, on the grounds that prostitutes could then be officially registered and required to submit to regular health checks. Legislation already exists in Britain which allows local authorities to keep a person with AIDS in hospital if it is considered they are a risk to others.

In the United States, several states are considering introducing legislation allowing prostitutes to be tested upon conviction or as a condition of probation. In Nevada, where brothels are licensed and state-regulated, the public health department requires that women registered as prostitutes be tested every month. Any woman who tests positive is denied employment as a prostitute. No one has suggested that all men who visit prostitutes be tested.

There have also been a number of proposals introduced which would make it a crime for someone who is antibody-positive to have sex with someone else. Whilst this could apply to many people, such proposals have been particularly aimed at prostitutes. In Florida, for instance, it is a misdemeanour for anyone who tests positive and has been informed of the result to engage in prostitution.

Clearly if prostitution is your main source of income it will be hard to stop. In parts of West Germany prostitutes who test positive are being advised of retraining programmes and other jobs available to them. Rather than introducing new forms of legal control of prostitutes, similar programmes in this country would help prostitutes who want to change their occupation to do so.

Rape

The fear of being raped is a form of male oppression all women share. It is something which, in countless ways, shapes our daily lives: whether we feel able to go out alone, especially at night; whether we feel dependent on a man for protection; whether we feel we could ever live alone. Recent statistics on sexual violence towards women confirm that this is a well-founded fear. Since 1980 the number of rapes in the UK has increased by 100 per cent. This reflects a steady increase in sexual offences against women in the last ten years. This may in part be due to women being more willing to report rape or to changes in police practice. But it undoubtedly represents the tip of the iceberg. In 1987, in England and Wales, there were more than 13,000 cases of indecent assault on women and girls reported and 2,471 cases of rape (Home Office figures). The real figure is likely to be much higher, if one takes into account the sexual violence that goes unreported and the extent of rape within marriage. According to British law, it is impossible for a woman to be raped by her husband. The rationale behind such laws is that marriage gives a man the right to sexual intercourse with his wife. This in turn stems from the idea that, once married, women are the property of their husbands.

The law further ignores women's experience of sexual violence by limiting its definition of rape to penetration of the vagina by a penis. Other forms of sexual violence, such as forced oral sex or anal intercourse, or the insertion of bottles, sticks or other objects into the vagina, however violent or humiliating, are not defined as rape. For the many women who have encountered sexual violence at some point in their lives, rape is the experience of being forced, against their will, to engage in sexual acts, which may include vaginal intercourse.

With AIDS, the fear of being raped takes on a new dimension. The rapist may be infected with HIV which may be transmitted during forced intercourse with a woman. The more violent the attack the more likely it is that a woman will suffer internal bruising, lacerations and bleeding. This may make it easier for the virus to enter the bloodstream.

A woman could say that she herself has AIDS or is infected with HIV as a means of trying to prevent rape. Whilst this might work in some situations it could also provoke more violence in others. Alternatively, fear of getting AIDS may not lead to a decrease in rape but may in future involve rapists using condoms, or other forms of sexual violence besides intercourse.

A common belief about rape is that it takes place between people who do not know each other. This is very often not the case. Many women are raped by their partners or dates or other acquaintances. Similarly, when children are sexually abused it is usually not by strangers but by a male relative or family 'friend' – men who have power over the child which they can use to force or persuade a child to have sex with them. While information on actual incidents of sexual abuse of children is, like rape, limited, it is estimated that 50,000 cases of sexual assault on female children take place every year in the UK. The fears we have for children in circumstances like this are increased by AIDS. Children may be penetrated vaginally, anally or orally. This will usually cause severe physical damage and a great deal of pain. If the man is infected with HIV, or other sexually transmitted diseases, transmission to the child could occur.

In some cases sexual violence against women and children leads to their death either from suicide, as a result of the emotional trauma caused by the attack, or from the physical injuries directly inflicted on them. Now there is a further possibility to consider: AIDS.

Whether or not she is infected with HIV, the worry that she may have been will, for some women, add to the trauma of rape. They will feel frightened about getting AIDS. They may worry about infecting others yet, in some cases, feel too afraid to tell their partners in case they might leave them or become violent. They may even have to deal with the possibility that it was not the rapist who infected them but their own partner. With rape, there is also the risk of pregnancy to consider. In those cases of pregnancy which are not terminated, if a woman was infected, the virus could be transmitted to the foetus. Pregnancy could also possibly increase a woman's own chances of developing AIDS.

These are difficult and complex issues to deal with in

conjunction with the emotional after-effects of rape. In future, rape crisis centres will need to consider these, and provide support services for women who have been raped and are considering taking the antibody test.

African women

It is estimated that in Africa women make up approximately half of the known number of AIDS cases. (As of October 1988, 19,141 cases of AIDS in Africa were reported to the W.H.O.) Many of these women are natives of Zaire or other Central African countries such as Kenya, Zambia and Uganda, where AIDS is known locally as 'slim disease' because of its association with weight loss.

The number of women infected with HIV is difficult to estimate, although figures commonly reported of one in ten people being infected with the virus in Central Africa are exaggerated. (See p. 8.)

How is HIV transmitted in Africa? Most Africans deny either injecting drugs or homosexual activity. Similarly, although some cases of AIDS have resulted from blood transfusions, the majority of African people with AIDS deny exposure to blood products. The suggestion that blood-sucking insects such as mosquitoes might be responsible for carrying the virus from person to person has now been dismissed. If this were the case one would expect AIDS to occur in all age groups and especially among children or rural workers who work outdoors and are more likely to be bitten. Instead, AIDS in Africa occurs mainly in people who are sexually active and who live in urban, not rural districts.

In the United States a study was conducted in Belle Glade, Florida to examine the likelihood of transmission of HIV by insects. This area was chosen because of its high number of AIDS cases and because these cases are primarily heterosexual. The study found no evidence of transmission of HIV by mosquitoes or other blood-sucking insects. What it did show was that HIV in Belle Glade is passed on mainly through contaminated needles and sexual contact.

Studies suggest that heterosexual activity, blood transfusions, transmission from mother to infant, and probably unsterilised needles, account for the occurrence of AIDS in Africa. While some do, not all African countries have the resources to screen blood donors for HIV antibodies. Also, the use of unsterilised needles for injecting vaccines and medicines is a common practice in parts of Africa, especially in poorer areas where, because of lack of equipment, one needle may be used to inject several people. The possibility that HIV may be passed on in this way, as well as through unscreened blood donations, has particular implications for women and children. Women often require blood transfusions during childbirth on account of anaemia resulting from multiple pregnancies or malaria. Children too often need blood transfusions against malarial anaemia, and vaccinations are frequently carried out by means of re-usable needles which are not always properly sterilised. (Transmission would also be possible through non-sterile instruments used for tattooing, ritual scarification, ear-piercing, circumcision, clitoridectomy and infibulation.)

It is generally believed that in Africa the main way in which AIDS is spread is by heterosexual activity. Anal intercourse, perhaps practised as a method of contraception, might be one way the virus is transmitted. (Anal intercourse may also occur as a result of cultural taboos about having vaginal sex whilst a woman is menstruating.) What most people say is that they don't have anal sex. This is not surprising. People are unlikely to want to admit they do things which are heavily stigmatised in their culture. Likewise, most Africans deny having oral sex or oral-anal contact. It is in the light of this, rather than of any detailed research on the rates of transmission associated with different sex acts, which in any case would be extremely difficult to carry out, that vaginal intercourse has come to be regarded as a major risk factor for African women.

It is important to remember that in parts of Africa many women are undernourished and in ill-health and consequently have suppressed immune systems. If co-factors are involved in the development of AIDS this may be a further risk factor. Also, the chances of a woman becoming infected with HIV are likely to be enhanced by the fact that in Africa untreated sexually transmitted diseases are more widespread. (It has been reported that up to 70 per cent of people seeking treatment in STD clinics in Africa are seen because of genital ulcers, as compared to about 4 per cent in the United States.) A woman who has a sexually transmitted infection such as gonorrhoea, for example, may have genital sores or ulcers which could make it easier for the virus to enter her bloodstream during intercourse. Many African studies do show an association between genital ulcers in women and HIV infection.

In addition to genital ulcers, a woman may also have open wounds as a result of clitoridectomy and infibulation (see Glossary) which are practised on a large number of African women. The most extreme form of female circumcision, *infibulation*, is the complete removal of the vulval tissue including the clitoris and labia. The sides of the wounds are then sewn together, leaving a minute opening. Vaginal intercourse is impossible unless the vagina is reopened, causing bleeding and lesions in the vaginal tissue which would allow easier transmission of semen containing the virus. That some African women may be at risk of AIDS as a result of female circumcision is another reason why those African governments who have not yet done so need to take urgent action to eradicate this practice.

The infections that a woman with AIDS will get will to some extent reflect the organisms already present in her body. These will vary according to where she has lived and the kind of life she has led. In the United States and Europe, for instance, about half of all those who have AIDS develop pneumocystis carinii pneumonia. This does not appear to be a common infection in African women with

AIDS; more likely they will develop re-activated infections such as tuberculosis.

Having many different sexual partners has also been suggested as a particular risk factor. The racist stereotyping of black people as sexually 'promiscuous' has a long history. But in this case it is black women's so called 'promiscuous' behaviour which has attracted most attention. In Africa, as elsewhere, it is women working as prostitutes who have been singled out and blamed for the 'spread' of infection.

In contrast to the United States and Europe, where it seems that unless a prostitute injects drugs infection with HIV is unusual, a large proportion of prostitutes in Central Africa are thought to be infected with the virus. In one study of Rwandan prostitutes living in the town of Butare, 29 of the 33 women tested had antibodies to the virus. Following on from this it has been suggested, though not proven, that many men who are infected with HIV in Africa are likely to have contracted the virus from prostitutes. But there is another way of looking at this. Since the virus can be transmitted to women through sexual contact with HIV infected men, prostitutes could be infected by their male customers – a possibility which many prostitutes fear.

Clearly AIDS is an important issue for African women. Over the next few years lots of African women will die from it and many more will become ill. Many of the children born to women with AIDS, or who are infected with HIV, will also die.

This situation will not change unless efforts are made to try and control the spread of the disease. Rather than seeking to pin the blame on someone, what is needed is that governments act quickly by adopting a widescale policy of AIDS prevention through major educational and public information programmes. Many countries in Africa have developed educational programmes, and did so before some Western states. But in some parts of Africa, this is made very difficult by a lack of resources and personnel to implement such programmes. Similarly, the health services may be ill-equipped to deal with halting the spread of the disease. In some African countries the funds simply aren't there, for instance, to screen blood donors routinely. The cost of an HIV antibody test is more than the amount of money allocated per head for a whole year's health care. Lack of money also means that in many parts of Africa the treatment for AIDS is restricted. This is a situation that is compounded by the fact that, in Africa, AIDS is just one of a number of important health issues. In Zambia, for example, thousands die each year of malaria; and millions of children die each year in Africa as a result of conditions linked to malnutrition.

As the social and economic consequences of AIDS in Africa become more apparent, it is to be hoped that other countries will support the development of health and educational services within Africa aimed at controlling the spread of the disease.

Haitian women

The first cases of AIDS were diagnosed among Haitians in the United States in mid 1982. At first, doctors claimed not to understand why people of Haitian descent were developing AIDS. Studies reported that homosexuality, injecting drug use and blood products did not appear to play major roles in the transmission of HIV among Haitians. This led to speculation that the virus might be transmitted through sharing needles to inject medicinal agents, or by some other, as yet unidentified, mode of transmission.

More recent research suggests that this 'mystery' was most likely the result of American doctors' inexperience in obtaining sensitive information. For instance, the strong social stigma attached to homosexuality within the Haitian community means that many Haitian men will be reluctant to say that they have had sex with other men.

In Haiti itself it would appear that, as the epidemic has progressed, there have been changes in the way in which the virus is transmitted. In 1983 the pattern of AIDS in Haiti resembled that in the United States – with many more men than women affected and the majority of cases attributed to homosexual contact or IV drug use. Now, there are signs that a similar picture to Africa is emerging with almost three-quarters of AIDS cases in Haiti believed to be caused by heterosexual contact. This is evidenced by the dramatic increase in the number of cases of women with AIDS over the last few years.

It was the initial inability of doctors to explain why Haitians were developing AIDS that led to their being categorised as a 'high-risk group'. What this implied was that it was something about Haitians, or their lifestyle, which put them at risk. This connection between AIDS and Haitians was also strengthened by the common, though unsubstantiated, belief that AIDS originated in Africa and spread to the rest of the world via Haiti. It is suggested that Haitians, working in Zaire and subsequently returning home, exported the HIV virus to Haiti, where visiting American tourists, most especially gay men, became infected. Such associations have been strongly resisted by Haitians themselves, who have condemned as racist the belief that AIDS is a Haitian disease. Certainly within the United States one consequence of classifying Haitians as high-risk for AIDS was an enhancement of the social and economic discrimination that many Haitians already faced. The Haitian government, concerned also about effects of such claims on Haiti's important tourist industry, demanded that Haitians be removed from the official list of groups at risk. This was finally achieved in 1985, when the CDC dropped Haitians from their list of risk groups.

Their action is supported by studies of the presence of HIV among Haitians. The rate of infection among the Haitian population is low. Simply being Haitian, in isolation from other risk factors, does not increase the risk of being infected with HIV. Despite this, AIDS-related discrimination still occurs. In New York, Haitian community workers claim that the fear of catching AIDS, though unfounded, has made it much harder for Haitians to find a job. Particularly hard-hit have been domestic workers, many of whom are women.

Blood transfusions

Very few people have contracted AIDS through blood transfusions. In Australia 5 per cent of the 943 cases of AIDS reported by August 1988 had been transfused with infected blood – most of them in New South Wales. In the United States over 75,000 cases of AIDS have been reported to the CDC (October 1988). Only 3 per cent of these were recipients of blood transfusions.

Though the risk is still low, the percentage is higher for women. As of October 1988, 6,260 women in the United States had AIDS. Of these, about 11 per cent had developed the disease following transfusion with blood or plasma which had been infected with HIV. In the UK thirteen women have been reported as having got AIDS this way (ten through transfusions received whilst abroad).

Although the numbers are not high, some women may still be worried about the possibility of getting AIDS through blood transfusions. This is perhaps not surprising given what they may have heard or read about AIDS. The widespread and, very often, sensationalised coverage of such cases by certain sections of the media has greatly exaggerated the risk of developing AIDS through transfusion. As a result of the introduction of screening procedures by blood banks, the chances of contracting HIV in this way in future are *extremely* small. If a transfusion is medically necessary the risks of not getting the transfusion are much higher than the risk of getting AIDS from the transfusion.

There also will be women, especially if they are planning a pregnancy, who are worried about past transfusions. In some countries, Australia for example, people who received a blood transfusion after 1980 are being recalled. If, despite the very low risk of infection, you decide to be tested, be sure to discuss the pros and cons beforehand (see pages 168–74).

Some women may also be worried about giving blood, in case it puts them at risk of getting AIDS through shared needles. The process of giving blood is not and never has been risky. All the equipment at blood donation centres is sterilised and used once only.

Before the introduction of screening procedures people were asked not to donate blood if they belonged to a high-risk group. As this mainly applied to men one suggestion put forward was that women only should be donors. The problem with this is that women can also have the virus. Another suggestion was that people could store their own blood until such time as they needed it. The advantage of using your own blood is that you won't receive anything from it that you didn't have already, including HIV.

Even with the introduction of screening some people are banking their own blood. The worry they have is that because of the gap between infection with the virus and the production of antibodies, some people who are infected will be undetected. In fact, the risk of this happening is extremely small: it is estimated that it might occur less than once in a million donations. Also, storing your own blood is only practical for planned operations and for people who are healthy enough and can afford to do so.

Since October 1985 in Britain and May 1985 in Australia, with the aim of making blood transfusions as safe as possible, it has been routine for all donated blood to be tested for HIV antibodies. (In view of the fact that the test occasionally produces false negatives, those in recognised risk groups are still being advised not to give blood.) Any blood found to be infected with HIV is rejected. Unfortunately this is not the case everywhere. In some countries the lack of effective screening of donors means that the transmission of HIV through blood transfusions will continue to occur.

One possible consequence of routinely testing donated blood is that some people might discover that they have been infected with HIV who would otherwise not have known. For most people this will be frightening news, and they will need access to support and counselling about what a positive test result means. Fortunately, the chances of this happening are extremely small. In the first six months during which it introduced screening the National Blood Transfusion Service tested over 845,000 women and men, all of whom had been asked not to give blood if they were in a 'high-risk' group. Out of these 845,000 only 16 were confirmed as antibody positive, and most of these were subsequently found to have been at risk either through sharing equipment to inject drugs or through sexual contact.

So, *unless* you or your sexual partner behave in ways that may put you at risk for infection there is no reason to fear finding out that you have the virus which can lead to AIDS, and it is safe to give blood.

Pregnancy

It is estimated that over 5,000 women in the United Kingdom may be infected with HIV (October 1988). Not all of these women will either want or be able to have children. However, for those who do desire motherhood the possible risks of pregnancy, both to themselves and to their potential offspring, need explaining.

Some researchers have suggested that pregnancy might increase an infected woman's chances of developing AIDS. But this has not been proven. More research needs to be done to determine whether this is the case and, if so, why. Hormonal changes that occur during pregnancy, or the fact that in a pregnant woman the immune system is suppressed to stop the body rejecting the foetus, have been suggested as possible explanations of why this might be the case.

If either you or your partner are at risk of becoming infected with HIV and are considering pregnancy (or if you find out that you are pregnant) it is important that *both* of you consider taking the antibody test. However you should only take the test after a full discussion of what the test results mean and the implications that may follow from a positive result. This will include being told that there is a high chance that the virus will be passed on to any children you might have.

If you test negative and your partner tests positive you might want to consider having a baby by artificial insemi-nation by donor, as the virus may be passed on from him to you during intercourse. Similarly, a woman who is already pregnant and is antibody negative should either avoid intercourse or use a condom if her male partner is positive. Otherwise she could contract the virus from him and, possibly, transmit it to the baby.

How this occurs is not entirely clear. At first it was thought that the virus was probably transmitted through the baby coming into contact with the mother's blood at or around the time of birth. Now we know that a pregnant woman who is infected with HIV can transmit it to the foetus. In one case cells infected with HIV were found in the tissues of a child born by caesarian section at 28 weeks to a woman who died of AIDS a few hours afterwards. The child also died three weeks later. Since the child was born by caesarean section and had no contact with his mother after delivery, this strongly suggests that the virus was passed on from mother to baby during pregnancy, via the placenta.

How likely this is, and when during pregnancy the virus travels across the placenta from mother to foetus, is also not clear. From the studies that have so far been done it is thought that there is a relatively high risk – estimated between a 25 to 40 per cent chance – of an infected mother giving birth to an infected child. The probability of trans-mission may be related to the length of time a woman has been infected or whether she has developed HIV-related illness. Others have suggested that the risk of transmission may be greater the more children a woman has, but this is not yet clear. What does seem likely is that a high proportion of HIV infected babies will go on to develop AIDS or other HIV-related illness. Many quickly become sick and, in addition to immune problems, may suffer damage to the brain and the nervous system.

Whereas amniocentesis can sometimes provide a woman with information that may help her to decide whether or not to have an abortion (for example, in the case of women at risk of having a child with Down's Syndrome) this is not the case in this situation. Transmission of the virus might occur at a later stage of pregnancy, after amniocentesis had been carried out, or at birth. Even then there is no way of telling if the baby is infected. This is because during the first year there is no way of knowing for certain whether antibodies produced to HIV are the infant's own or have been passed on from the mother. Whilst not all women will be aware that they could have infected their infant, for those who are this period of uncertainty is likely to be extremely stressful.

Because of the possible risks to both mother and baby surrogacy arrangements have been affected by AIDS. The possibility that the surrogate mother, if infected, could pass the HIV virus on to the child is likely to lead to surrogates being tested for HIV antibodies. The father should also be tested. Otherwise the surrogate could contract the virus from him and become ill, as well as possibly transmitting it to the baby.

At present the number of infants with AIDS is extremely small relative to the total number of people with AIDS. By October 1988 there were 1,202 cases of AIDS in children in the United States out of a total of 75,768. Similarly, in Britain and Australia AIDS in infants accounts for only about 1 per cent of all reported cases. This may change, of course, as the number of women who have been infected with HIV gradually increases.

There is a handful of cases worldwide where a child is

thought to have become infected with HIV through breast-milk. In one case a woman gave birth by caesarean section. Because of blood loss during the operation, she was given a blood transfusion after delivery. The baby, a boy, survived and was subsequently breastfed by her. Later it was discovered that the blood used in the transfusion had been donated by someone who had since gone on to develop AIDS. Both mother and baby were tested and found to have antibodies to HIV. As the mother was apparently infected after delivery, transmission of the virus to the child could not have occurred at birth or during pregnancy. It was suggested that the child became infected with HIV through the mother's milk.

To avoid this possible risk to the infant, women known to be HIV antibody positive, or at risk of HIV infection, are being discouraged from breastfeeding (although it is acknowledged that this advice may need to change in the light of new knowledge). It has also been recommended that they do not give milk to milk banks. Many hospitals run breast milk banks. Women who produce more milk than their own babies need donate the surplus, which is then given to premature babies and babies with bowel disorders. Breast milk banks in the UK are now pasteurising donated breast milk which destroys the virus – though this also damages some of its anti-infective properties. The Department of Health also recommends that donors should be known to be HIV antibody negative.

Studies need to be done to establish whether breastfeeding can transmit the virus. It may turn out to be very important that potentially infected babies *are* breastfed. In terms of its nutritional value and anti-infective properties breast milk is better than artificial milk. Another concern is that baby milk companies will use the fact that HIV has been found in breast milk to promote their products. In countries where women cannot bottle feed safely, either because of the cost or access to adequate sanitation, such advice could put a child's life at greater risk than the possibility of HIV infection. In many developing countries bottle fed babies are much more likely to die than breast-fed babies.

Advice about the relationship between pregnancy and AIDS should be available to all women. Apart from public education campaigns, there is a need for well-informed and sensitive counselling services for women infected with HIV, or at risk of infection, who are considering pregnancy or are already pregnant. Similarly, women who are themselves healthy but have passed the virus on to their child are also likely to need the help and support of others in dealing with their feelings, very often, of guilt. Many women don't know, prior to their child being diagnosed with AIDS, that they are infected with HIV. This means that they are confronted with a number of extremely difficult issues at once: a child with AIDS, their own potential to develop the disease and the fact that they have passed the virus on to their child.

Most importantly, a woman should be able to talk to someone whom she feels is sympathetic and has an understanding of what she is going through. It's also important that counselling includes adequate and comprehensive advice about contraception and abortion. However this will only be useful if women also have access to them.

It is the medical profession which, to a large extent, controls women's access to contraception and abortion. Many doctors believe that wanting a baby is normal, instinctive and desirable in women, especially if they are married. Such beliefs have an important influence on medical practice, and can lead to a woman finding it difficult to get an abortion or certain forms of contraception. In the case of women who are infected with HIV, the medical advice is don't have children. Where a woman who is infected with the virus is already pregnant, the recommendation is that she be considered for, and counselled about, an abortion.

Whilst the relationship between pregnancy and AIDS may help to bring about improvements in services for women which are not specific to AIDS, such as better contraceptive advice, it could also lead to further restrictions in women's reproductive rights. For example, does a woman who is infected with the HIV virus have the right to begin or maintain a pregnancy? According to some, all women who test positive should be sterilised or, if they are already pregnant, be made to have an abortion. (Sterilisation may be seen as a 'solution', for instance, by those who oppose abortion.) This is in spite of the fact that not all babies born to sero-positive women are infected.

It has also been suggested that the HIV antibody test should be compulsory for all women who are pregnant. It is important for women to have access to safe, low cost or no cost abortion, and to proper education and counselling about taking the HIV antibody test – but this must be offered on a voluntary and not a forced basis. Women need to be told of the risks and supported in the decisions *they* make about whether to take the antibody test or, if they are pregnant, whether to have an abortion.

Some pregnant women who test positive do decide to have an abortion; others continue with the pregnancy. For some women, deciding not to have a child, whether this involves having an abortion or not, will be difficult. For many women becoming a mother is an important aspect of how she sees herself and her future, a view which society strongly encourages in the importance it places on women wanting and being able to have children, especially if they are married. For women addicted to using IV drugs, pregnancy may be one of the few times they feel good about themselves, and have an incentive to change their drug-taking behaviour. They may feel accepted, as almost 'normal', a 'real' woman. Weighing the risk of an infected child against the rejection they may have felt by society, it is easy to see how some may decide to continue with the pregnancy.

It's important also to consider the rights of women to make their own decisions about reproduction. For those who want an abortion this may not be an option either because abortion is illegal, as in Ireland for example, or difficult to get unless you are able to pay. There are also race issues to consider. It's one thing for a doctor to advise a white woman who is HIV antibody positive not to have children, it's another to say this to a black woman. Historically, black women have been subject to forced sterilisation and coerced family-planning decisions. For this reason it is essential that public health measures respect the autonomy of black women.

Apart from influencing how a woman who is infected with HIV may feel about 'choosing' not to have children, the pressures on women to become mothers may also affect the spread of AIDS. Women who want to get pregnant, unless they are using artificial insemination, will be engaging in vaginal intercourse. If either the woman or her male partner is infected with HIV then transmission of the virus to the uninfected partner may occur.

Remember, we are talking specifically about women who are either infected with HIV or who are at risk of infection.

Artificial insemination

Vaginal intercourse, though the most common method, is not the only way of getting pregnant. Each year thousands of babies are born as a result of artificial insemination by donor (AID). The reasons why women use artificial insemination vary. Some women use this method because they can't get pregnant by their partner. Others, who are not in a steady relationship, may feel that the time is right for them to have a child on their own. Artificial insemination has also been used by lesbians who wish to conceive a child without having sex with a man. Although this might sound strange to some, wanting to have sex with someone and wanting to have a child can be quite separate desires. Another reason why some lesbians may prefer to have an AID baby is to try to ensure undisputed guardianship and custody of their child. This is very understandable given the court's reluctance to grant custody, and sometimes access, to lesbian mothers.

With artificial insemination, a syringe and not a penis is used to introduce sperm deep into a woman's vagina. This is done around the time when a woman is ovulating. The whole procedure is simple, and some women carry it out themselves without the help of doctors or an official donor organisation. In this case the term self-insemination is used.

In recent years some lesbians, and other women who are interested in becoming pregnant through artificial insemination, have become concerned about the possibility of gettings AIDS. In November 1984, following publicity about AIDS, all artificial insemination clinics in Australia were closed. This decision was controversial, not only because artificial insemination was regarded as an important service for many infertile heterosexual couples, but also because there were no reported cases of AIDS due to donor insemination. In 1985, however, four Australian women who had been artificially inseminated were found to have antibodies to HIV. They had all been inseminated with semen from a donor who was subsequently found to be infected with the virus. One of the women has since gone on to develop ARC.

This resulted in many clinics having to discard samples of donated sperm, where past donors could not be located and tested for antibodies to HIV. This is a procedure which has since been repeated both here and in the United States.

Women planning donor insemination should not be alarmed by this. They do however need to know what the risks are and what precautions they should take. Basically you should make sure that the donor you are using has not been infected by HIV. At the moment this is determined by the HIV antibody test. Those who test positive will most likely still be infected with the virus and will be capable of passing it on if they donate semen. A negative result to the test *usually* means that the person is not infected. Occasionally, however, the test produces false negatives. For this reason some women may decide not to use semen from men who may be at risk, even if they have a negative antibody test. This includes gay or bisexual men who engage in 'unsafe' sex, men who share equipment to inject drugs and some haemophiliacs.

Since the beginning of 1985, most clinics offering artificial insemination have tested prospective donors for infection with HIV. If you are inseminating through a clinic be sure to ask if the donor's blood has been properly tested for HIV. You should insist on *frozen* sperm, preferably from a clinic that does not use sperm until the donor has been tested a second time a few months later. This is because in the early stages of infection the body does not produce antibodies to HIV. This means that if someone were tested shortly after having been infected the test would be negative. Retesting after a few months would solve this. In Australia, many sperm banks have a holding and retesting period of six months.

Women doing self-insemination also need to be careful in choosing a donor. In the past gay men have often acted as donors. Now, with a large number of gay men thought to be infected with the virus, especially in the London area, gay men are being advised not to donate sperm and it would seem safest not to use them as donors if they engage in high-risk behaviours. Similarly, men who are not gay or bisexual should not act as donors if they engage in activities that put them at risk of infection such as, for instance, injecting drugs and sharing needles.

Whoever your donor is you should make every attempt to find out how likely it is that he may be infected with HIV. Apart from being asked detailed questions about his medical, social and sexual background, he should have the HIV antibody test. For reasons I have already outlined, this would involve his taking the test twice, with at least a three-month gap between tests. If both tests were negative, the sperm could be used *providing* that the donor had done nothing to put himself at risk of infection in the period between the first and second test. Otherwise there would be no knowing if the second negative result would, in a few months time, become positive. This is a worry for some women, especially if they don't feel they can trust their donor completely. One solution is to have the donor's sperm frozen at a sperm bank while waiting for the results of the second test. However some women, because of financial or other reasons, may not have access to a sperm bank.

Some women who have used donors who fall into a category labelled 'high-risk', or who inseminated before 1985 when screening was introduced, may be worried about the possibility of being infected and developing AIDS. (This applies also to women who have attempted to become pregnant via AID and failed, using untested sperm.) This is extremely unlikely. No cases of AIDS or other HIV-related illness due to artificial insemination have so far been reported in this country or in the United States. It is possible to find out if you have been infected with HIV by having the antibody test. However this is something you should think very carefully about before doing. If you are extremely anxious or worried about the possibility of being infected with HIV, especially if you are considering pregnancy, then it may help to have the test. On the other hand if you do have the test you must be fully prepared to accept that it might turn out to be positive, a result which could have serious emotional and practical consequences. For women who are worried about whether they may be infected some of the pros and cons of taking the test are discussed in Chapter Seven.

3 Lesbians and AIDS

What does AIDS have to do with lesbians? This is a question which you could be forgiven for asking. After all, very few lesbians are known to have developed AIDS and, generally speaking, lesbians are considered to be at low-risk for AIDS and other sexually transmitted diseases.

Nevertheless, AIDS does affect lesbians, both personally and politically, in a number of ways. As health care workers and as workers in AIDS projects, lesbians are involved in the care of people with AIDS. Some lesbians have been affected by AIDS-related deaths or illnesses of gay men they know. Others who are ill-informed about the disease may be anxious about going to mixed gay clubs or bars because they are afraid they might get AIDS. Lesbians are also affected by the strengthening of homophobia and anti-lesbianism which the disease or, more accurately, its portrayal in the mass media has led to. The association of the fear of AIDS with the fear of homosexuality may affect the rights of lesbians, as well as gay men, in areas of housing, employment, insurance cover, etc. In particular lesbians may experience greater violence towards them because of AIDS. Also of concern to lesbians are the problems that AIDS raises for those considering artificial insemination. Finally, lesbians are involved because, like other women, they too can get AIDS.

The main impact of AIDS on the lesbian community relates to the way in which AIDS has been seen, wrongly, as a 'gay disease' *and* the way in which lesbians have been categorised together with gay men. This has led to lesbians being labelled in some people's minds as at risk for AIDS. One consequence of this is that some lesbians have been refused as blood donors on the grounds that their 'homosexuality' puts them at risk.

In 1986, Nottingham Blood Transfusion Service refused to accept a woman's blood after she told them she was a lesbian. Shortly afterwards she received a letter stating the Services policy of not accepting lesbian blood, because of the supposed risk of it being infected with HIV. In response to this, Nottingham Lesbian Line campaigned and were successful in getting this policy changed on the grounds that lesbians are probably least at risk of AIDS.

The importance of making it clear that lesbianism is the safest sexuality around at present is not only to counter the homophobia generated by the fear of AIDS. It also highlights an inherent contradiction in the idea that AIDS is God's punishment for 'homosexuality'. By this reasoning, if AIDS proves that certain acts are morally wrong then God must be a lesbian!

Asserting our visibility as lesbians is also important at a time when widespread fear of AIDS may lead to attempts to restrict certain sexual practices. A good example of this is Section 28 of the 1988 Local Government Act which bans local authorities from 'promoting homosexuality' and forbids the teaching of the 'acceptability of homosexuality as a pretended family relationship'. This law will legitimise the prejudices of those who want nothing to do with lesbians and gay men. Even before the Section became law it was being used as an excuse to discriminate against lesbians and gays.

Many lesbians have been insulted and threatened in connection with AIDS. Increased anti-gay hostility and discrimination as a result of the ignorance and hysteria which surround AIDS can affect lesbians in other ways. The reluctance of the courts to grant custody and, in some cases, access to lesbian mothers is well known. Behind these actions lies the assumption that lesbians do not make good mothers. This is very often based on a concern that children of a lesbian mother will grow up to be lesbian or gay themselves. This is a view which is not only discriminatory, in regarding being lesbian or gay as an undesirable outcome, but is also without foundation. More recently, a new objection to lesbian motherhood has emerged. In the United States, a lesbian mother was denied visitation rights because of the judge's fear that she might give her children AIDS.

Historically there has been tension between the lesbian community and gay men. Nevertheless, many lesbians, especially in the United States, have played an important role in the development of AIDS organisations, fundraising and other forms of AIDS-related work. One example of lesbian involvement was the 'Our Brothers Need Blood' campaign in San Francisco. This, and similar campaigns in other American cities, was aimed at getting lesbians to donate blood in support of gay men. Women donated blood and credited their blood units to a special account, available to people with AIDS in need of blood. The account was established to alleviate some of the costs incurred during a transfusion. A situation that is made more difficult by the fact that many health insurance companies are reluctant to provide cover for gay men, especially if they are antibody positive, because they are perceived as high-risk for AIDS.

For some lesbians the primary motive for doing AIDS-work has been a political one. They see increased homophobia as affecting the lesbian community and feel that fighting AIDS discrimination *is* a lesbian issue. Other lesbians have become involved in AIDS work because AIDS has affected them personally, as well as politically, through the death of women they know or gay male friends.

Equally, there are lesbians who, whilst they may sympathise with gay men over AIDS, believe it is important that they put their time and energy into issues which they feel are of more direct relevance to women and, more especially, to other lesbians. Some lesbians feel angry that gay men, who have previously shown little interest or involvement in issues that concern women, now expect lesbians to support them.

Such reactions are perhaps more likely among lesbians living in the UK than in America, where there is a stronger tradition of lesbians and gay men working together in 'mixed' organisations; although some lesbians in the United States have also asked themselves 'Would gay men be there for lesbians if AIDS had happened to us?' A question that is borne out by the fact that encountering sexism from the gay men they work with would seem to be an all too common experience for women working in AIDS organisations.

It is not necessary to feel any political affinity with gay men to become involved in AIDS work. For example, some lesbians have become involved because they are concerned about the way AIDS is affecting other women, especially in relation to reproductive rights.

A tension also exists between the lesbian and gay community and those who identify themselves as bisexual. Previously, some lesbians have argued that bisexuals are sheltered under a label of comparative privilege. A woman who identifies herself as bisexual can have sexual relationships with other women without experiencing the same degree of social rejection that would be involved in a commitment to a lesbian identity. Now, with AIDS, some lesbians are also concerned that bisexual women may pass on HIV to the lesbian community. What it is important to realise is that risk of infection comes from what you do, now how you define yourself.

Who is at risk?

No one knows exactly how many lesbians have AIDS or have died from HIV-related illness. This is not only because some women who have got AIDS may not want to say that they are lesbians. Unlike cases of AIDS in men, women with AIDS are not classified according to their sexual preference. This is perhaps not surprising, given the lack of medical recognition of lesbian health issues in general.

A small number of AIDS in women identified as lesbian have been officially reported to the CDC, in the United States – these were either due to IV drug use or the result of a blood transfusion. The reported cases represent only those women who have been diagnosed as having AIDS and who are also known to be lesbian. Informal reporting of lesbians with AIDS suggests that the unofficial figure may be somewhat higher, primarily as a result of sharing equipment to inject drugs. The San Francisco AIDS Foundation, for example, reports that of the few lesbians they know who have AIDS most fall into the category of injecting drug user.

Although accurate figures are not available, the CDC, the organisation that is monitoring the AIDS epidemic in the United States, considers lesbians to be the lowest 'risk group' for AIDS. Consequently, most lesbians need worry very little about getting AIDS. Because of this we need to be very careful, in talking about lesbians and AIDS, not to create anxieties but rather to emphasise that many, if not most, lesbians are not at risk. At the same time, lesbians should not see themselves as immune to the disease. *Anyone* can become infected with HIV given the relevant risk factors.

That some people have assumed that lesbians don't get AIDS is interesting. It tells us a great deal about the way we define someone as lesbian. It begs the question 'What is a lesbian?.' (It also raises questions about what is lesbian sex?)

Some lesbians may occasionally have sex with men who may be at risk. Some lesbians who now only have sex with women used to have sex with men before they became a lesbian. Some lesbians inject drugs and share equipment to do so. Some lesbians are prostitutes who under pressure, either from a pimp or for economic reasons, may be forced to agree to have intercourse with male clients without using a condom. A growing number of lesbians are parents either as a result of artificial insemination or through sexual intercourse with a man. Lesbians, too, are sexually abused and raped.

A lesbian is at risk of HIV infection, as is any woman, only to the extent of her risky behaviour. It's important to remember this. Just because you call yourself a lesbian doesn't mean that you won't become infected if you have unsafe sex with men who could have the virus, or share equipment to inject drugs. With AIDS, the risk comes from what you do not how you label yourself. That's why it's important to discuss behaviours, rather than what a person identifies as. In this sense, it's more appropriate to talk of the risks to women who have sex with other women than the risks of 'lesbian sex'. However, we also need to recognise that lesbians are a distinct social group, with a certain identity and history of discrimination which AIDS has revitalised. While it may make more sense in terms of transmission to talk of sex between women, in terms of the social and political issues surrounding AIDS it is important that we recognise how *lesbians*, as a group, are affected.

It is lesbians who share needles or other equipment for mixing and injecting drugs who run the biggest risk of contracting HIV. This is one of the many reasons why substance abuse among lesbians needs to be more openly talked about. Of the very few cases of AIDS among lesbians that have been reported in the United States, most have a history of injecting drug use. To date, there have been no studies done which deal specifically with the incidence of IV drug use among lesbians. In San Francisco, the Lesbian AIDS Project is currently looking at the rate of infection among (self-identified) lesbian IV drug users.

Lesbians are also at risk if they engage in unsafe sex with men who are at risk. As various studies have shown, there is no necessary association between regarding yourself as a lesbian and only having sex with women. Some lesbians do have sex with men. Nevertheless, many women do choose to have sexual relationships only with women. They, and

---

Lesbians are at risk of being infected with HIV if they:

- Share needles or any other equipment for injecting and mixing drugs.
- Have had unsafe sex with men at risk some time over the last nine years.
- Have used semen for artificial insemination from a donor who is infected with HIV.
- Have received blood transfusions or blood products with blood infected with HIV between 1979 and 1985. (In the UK and in the United States this risk has largely been eliminated, since 1985, through the introduction of screening of blood.)
- Have had unsafe sex with women who have the virus.

---

other lesbians who decide that they want a child by artificial insemination, may be at risk if they use a donor who is infected. In addition to the risk to themselves there is also the possibility, if they do become infected with HIV, that the virus could be passed on to any child they might have. (Assessing the risk of artificial insemination is discussed in more detail on pages 64–67).

Since most clinics now screen would-be donors for HIV infection, this particularly applies to women who are carrying out insemination for themselves, without the help of an official donor organisation. There are several reasons why some lesbians may prefer to do this. First of all it allows a woman a greater amount of control over the process of insemination. (Though some lesbians have been successful in obtaining artificial insemination on the National Health Service, the medical profession generally regards artificial insemination as a way of helping heterosexual couples conceive a child.) It also means that she can choose a known donor. Choosing a known or an unknown donor can be a complex decision and, while many do not, some women may want their child to know the father. Also, the cost of using a sperm bank may be prohibitive for some women.

Insemination choices for lesbians have been limited because of AIDS. In the past, lesbians have often used gay men as donors. One of the advantages of this is that there would seem to be less likelihood of a gay man using a woman's lesbianism against her in a later dispute over the child. With the spread of AIDS, gay men have been advised not to donate blood or sperm. Although not all gay men are infected with HIV, or have engaged in high-risk behaviours, a high proportion are thought to be affected. Studies of gay men attending STD clinics in the London area indicate that 20 per cent are infected with the virus. Lesbians planning self-insemination should therefore think very carefully about using gay men, or indeed *any man who could be at risk*, as donors.

As a further safeguard it is important to get information about your donor's health, medical and sexual history. With the availability of the antibody test, many lesbians have also asked their donors to be tested. For the reasons which I have already outlined in the previous chapter, the antibody test should be done twice prior to insemination with a period of three to six months between tests. Your donor should practise safe sex between tests and should not engage in any other high-risk activities. If the second test is positive the donor's semen should not be used. If the test is negative then the semen will most probably be safe to use. Lesbians who plan to self-inseminate could ask to have the donor's sperm frozen at a sperm bank whilst waiting for a donor's follow-up test.

Research on the possible risk of infection with HIV through donor insemination is virtually non-existent. In San Francisco the Lesbian Insemination Project, a statewide study of lesbians who have been inseminated since 1979, is the first of its kind. (Since so many gay men in San Francisco are infected with the virus, and because many lesbians have used semen from gay men, questions about HIV infection have been critical for lesbians there.) In this ongoing study all the lesbians taking part are given the HIV antibody test and, in addition, are asked to complete a questionnaire about their insemination history. Many of the 80 or so women who have been interviewed – at least a third – used gay or bisexual men as donors. All of the women tested so far have been negative, including those who used donors who tested positive.

Research is only just beginning on how well the virus lives in menstrual blood or vaginal and cervical fluids, and no one knows definitely how or if women can sexually transmit HIV to other women. To ascertain this one would need to carry out studies of the female sexual partners of women who are antibody positive or who have AIDS. Needless to say, such studies are virtually non-existent.

There have, so far, been only two cases reported of possible transmission between two women through sexual contact. The first, reported in December 1986, involved a woman IV drug user who contracted the virus through sharing needles. She first developed symptoms of HIV infection, swollen lymph nodes and weight loss, in 1981. The following year she began a relationship with another woman who also developed swollen lymph nodes four to six weeks after their first sexual contact. In 1984 the first woman developed Kaposi's sarcoma and was subsequently found to be antibody positive. Her lover also tested positive.

Other than sexual contact, the second woman had no apparent risk factors for HIV infection. She denied ever having used IV drugs and had never had a blood transfusion. The conclusion drawn by the researchers was that the second woman contracted HIV from the first through sexual contact which included oral sex during the first woman's menstruation, oral-anal contact and vaginal sex that produced bleeding in both women.

Closer examination of this case reveals there were, however, other risk factors. The second woman had had sex with four other partners in the period between 1977 and being diagnosed as antibody positive in 1984 – including intercourse with a bisexual man with whom she had used a condom. Her other sexual contacts were with one woman and two heterosexual men, none of whom reported any risk factors. One man tested antibody negative, the other declined the test but reported that he was in excellent health.

The other case, reported in July 1987, is similarly lacking in detail. It involved a woman, born in the Philippines, who in 1986 discovered she was HIV antibody positive. She denied all heterosexual contact and IV drug use, and had no history of blood transfusion. However, during the previous five years she had had sex, including oral sex, with a number of different women.

Even if woman-to-woman transmission is possible it is, at present, extremely rare and the risk appears to be very low. This may be related to the mechanism by which HIV can be transmitted. For instance, we know that in the case of other sexually transmitted diseases while close genital contact is sufficient to contract herpes or genital warts, mucous membrane penetration facilitates transmission of diseases such as syphilis or gonorrhoea. It may also be harder for a woman to transmit HIV to another woman (or to a man) because the amount of infected vaginal/cervical secretions transferred during sex is less than the amount of infected semen transferred. Also, if few lesbians are infected at present then the odds are lower that HIV will be sexually transmitted by women to other women.

Nevertheless, until more is known about the possibility of woman-to-woman transmission, lesbians are being advised to follow safer sex guidelines if they think they, or their lover, may be at risk of infection.

Safer sex

As lesbians, we rarely talk about what we do in bed. This silence about sexual activities is an understandable reaction, given that it is the sexual aspects of being a lesbian that have tended to dominate how others see us. Another important reason is that sexual acts between women are very often interpreted as a 'turn on' for men, whether as pornography or not.

One of the consequences of not discussing our sex lives with other lesbians is that we often have to struggle alone, or with our lovers, in dealing with our sexual difficulties and worries. Breaking down the silence around lesbian sex is also important so that we can realistically assess what risks, if any, we are taking when it comes to sexually transmitted diseases such as AIDS.

It is important to re-emphasise, unless some lesbians become unnecessarily frightened or turned off sex, that most lesbians will have little reason to be concerned about getting AIDS, and will have no need to change their sexual behaviour. Those whose activities place them at risk of HIV infection, however, do need to take precautions. (Safer sex for women in heterosexual relationships is discussed in the following chapter.)

Concern about AIDS doesn't mean that you can't have sex. Rather, it means that you may have to change the type of sexual practices you enjoy, in situations where either you or your lover may be infected. This may be easier for lesbians than for women having sexual relations with men. Because the act of 'penetration' does not have the same meaning or significance for lesbian lovemaking as it does for heterosexual sex, a woman's female lover may be less likely to regard safer sex as dull or unexciting sex.

There are many ways in which women enjoy making love with one another. These include kissing on the mouth, kissing or caressing other parts of the body, touching or licking the clitoris and labia, stimulation of the breasts and nipples and rubbing against each other. Some women also like their vaginas to be touched at some point during lovemaking.

In recent years sado-masochistic (s/m) and other practices such as 'fist-fucking' have been the subject of heated controversy among lesbians. This is an important debate which deserves further discussion. Unfortunately, within the context of this book there is not the space to do justice to the arguments about why many lesbians object to such practices.

What activities put lesbians at risk for HIV infection? In order for infection to occur the virus must be transmitted into the bloodstream. Certain sexual practices and blood transfusion through shared needles allow that to happen. Therefore, if you believe that you or your partner may be infected with the virus, or you are not sure, you should avoid certain body fluids coming into contact with your mouth, rectum, vagina or any break in the skin through which the virus might gain entrance to the bloodstream. The body fluids you need to be especially concerned about are blood (including menstrual blood) and cervical and vaginal secretions. Although HIV has been found in saliva, there is no evidence that it can be transmitted this way.

The following are safer sex guidelines for lesbians who may be at risk of either getting or giving the virus through sexual contact. They are based on what we currently know about HIV transmission and may therefore change as more information becomes available.

Safe sex between women

There is little or no need to worry about becoming infected through:

- Hugging or massaging each other.
- Touching your own genitals (masturbation).
- Kissing. There is no evidence of HIV having been transmitted solely through exposure to saliva. The only time when kissing might transmit the virus would be through 'wet kissing', in which large amounts of saliva are passed. Provided neither partner has open cuts or sores of the mouth, lips or tongue, kissing probably represents little or no risk.
- Rubbing breasts together.
- Rubbing bodies together.
- Body kissing.

- Sharing sexual fantasies.
- Using vibrators, or other sex toys, providing that they are not shared or are protected with condoms, or are cleaned and dried thoroughly between each partner's use. Sex toys can be cleaned using household bleach diluted one part bleach to ten parts water. Make sure that the bleach solution is thoroughly washed off before use.
- Rubbing genitals on a partner's *unbroken* skin carries little or no risk of infection.
- Hand or finger-to-genital contact if there are no cuts or open sores on your hands. This includes activities such as 'mutual masturbation' and vaginal or anal 'penetration' with fingers. Putting fingers into the vagina of another woman whilst she is menstruating carries more risk. Uncut nails can cause tiny tears in the rectum and vagina so be sure fingernails are clipped. If you have cuts, scratches or sores on your fingers or hands, wearing disposable surgical rubber gloves will reduce the risk of coming into contact with infected blood or vaginal secretions. Alternatively, you could put a condom or finger cot on your finger(s). (Finger cots, condoms and latex gloves can be bought at chemists and from medical supply firms). Transmission is more probable from putting unprotected fingers into a woman's vagina or anus than from stimulation of the clitoris.
- Caressing and fondling each other.
- Touching a woman's breasts and nipples.
- Bathing together.
- Watching each other masturbate.
- Touching your own genitals at the same time as your lover touches hers.
- Sucking on the nipples of a woman (providing she is not lactating or otherwise secreting).
- Any activities that do not draw blood or involve body fluids which can transmit the virus coming into contact with body openings or breaks in the skin.

Unsafe sex might include

- Oral sex (or cunnilingus) is where one woman stimulates her lover's genitals with her mouth or tongue. Oral sex carries some risk to the woman 'going down on her lover', because there is a chance that the virus may be transmitted through vaginal fluids or, if she is menstruating, through a woman's menstrual blood. Open sores in the mouth make transmission more likely.

  Oral sex may be less risky if it is done using a thin piece of latex between the tongue and the vulva. You could use dental dams for this (thin rubber sheets available from dental supply companies) or, alternatively, cut a condom in half and use that. Condoms have the advantage of being easier to obtain and are usually thinner and more transparent than rubber dams. For some lesbians, however, the association of condoms with straight sex will be a turn off and, for this reason, they will be reluctant to use them.

  Many people may find latex barriers awkward to use. One solution is to make a pair of 'safe-sex pants'. Cut out the gusset of a pair of pants and fix a latex barrier in its place. That way the barrier stays put and your hands are free to touch your lover in other ways.

  Putting lubricant between the vulva and the barrier will increase sensation. Make sure it is a water-based lubricant, preferably one that contains nonoxynol-9 which is known to be effective against HIV. Oil-based lubricants destroy rubber. (See page 95 for a fuller discussion of nonoxynol-9 and lubricants.)

  Another way of reducing risk if a woman is menstruating is to use a diaphragm or cervical cap to prevent the flow of blood into the vagina. (This will not of course prevent contact with vaginal secretions, only menstrual blood.)

- Sex involving contact with urine – 'watersports' – might

be risky if urine gets in open cuts or body openings, since it may contain blood.

- Oral-anal contact (rimming). Apart from the other health risks associated with 'rimming', hepatitis B infection for instance, HIV may be transmitted by blood in faeces. Open sores in the mouth or bleeding gums make transmission more likely. Risk may be reduced by using a latex barrier.

- Rubbing genitals together could be risky because vaginal fluids may be exchanged and can enter tiny cuts and abrasions.

- Urine or faeces in the mouth or vagina.

- Sharing sex toys, such as vibrators, could be risky. As well as cleaning them thoroughly after use, putting a condom on vibrators or other sex toys if they are shared will help reduce the risk of infection. Use a new condom each time.

- Fisting (hand in rectum or vagina). Because the walls of the rectum and vagina can be easily injured during fisting the inserting partner's fingers or hand may be exposed to her partner's blood, bloody faeces or vaginal fluids. Using plenty of water-based lubricant and wearing disposable surgical rubber gloves reduces the risk.

- S/m activities causing bleeding. Any practice that breaks the skin or draws blood, either inside the vagina or anus or on the skin, puts you at risk of either giving (if you are infected) or getting (if you are not infected) the virus.

- Related to this, any type of blood-to-blood contact, including menstrual blood, is unsafe.

Lesbians who share equipment to inject drugs are also at risk for AIDS and should not share needles or other equipment for mixing and injecting drugs. The risks associated with injecting drug use and how to reduce them by coming off or changing the way you use drugs are discussed on pages 29–35.

A worry some lesbians may have – despite the fact that so very few lesbians have developed AIDS – is how to know whether their new lover is at risk? The simple answer is to ask. If you have a new sexual partner find out about her history and share your own. Do either of you, for instance, have a history of sharing equipment to inject drugs or having unsafe sex with men at risk? Telling other lesbians that you have slept with men, or that you inject drugs, can be a difficult thing to do. However, it is vital if you think you may be at risk that you let your partner(s) know. By talking it will be possible to realistically assess whether, like most lesbians, you are not at risk of either getting or giving HIV or, alternatively, you need to follow safer sex guidelines.

If you have sex with men, gay or straight, you should make every effort to find out if they are at risk of being infected with HIV and, if they are, follow the safer sex guidelines described in the following chapter. Remember, sexual intercourse with a man carries much more risk of getting AIDS and other sexually transmitted diseases than sex with another woman.

Lesbians with AIDS

Lesbians who get AIDS may experience special problems given that the health care system is designed for and administered by a predominantly heterosexual population. Staff may hold negative attitudes about lesbianism, making it difficult for lesbians to feel comfortable, especially in expressing physical affection towards their women friends and lovers. Similarly, some hospital regulations may discriminate against lesbians. Visiting rules, for example, may specify 'immediate family only'. Whilst you can put down who you like as next-of-kin, not all lesbians may be aware of this. This could cause a great deal of distress if hospital staff do not recognise that lesbians may regard their lovers as next-of-kin.

This may also apply when a woman dies from AIDS. The feelings one has when one's lover dies are no less painful for lesbians than for anyone else. What is different, often, is the context in which the process of mourning takes place. Lesbian relationships are not socially recognised or accepted in the same way that heterosexual or family relationships are. As a consequence of this a lesbian may not be invited to her lover's funeral and, if no will was made, may have to face the ordeal of her dead lover's family sharing out savings or possessions. This is one reason why it is important to make a will.

Clearly the process of mourning will be much more difficult for women who are isolated and have no one to talk to about how they feel. Even those lesbians who have the support of others may experience this to some degree, if, for example, they have not come out at work or to their family. Some lesbian and gay organisations provide practical help and emotional support to lesbians whose lovers have died. The gay bereavement project, for example, is a 24-hour service which can also give advice about making wills and funeral arrangements. They can be contacted through London Lesbian and Gay Switchboard, whose number is listed at the end of the book.

One of the problems in telling others that you are a lesbian is the hostile and violent reactions that this can evoke. It can also mean having to deal with rejection. For example, one of the problems lesbians have in coming out to their parents is that they may assume, wrongly, that this is somehow their 'fault'. Typically this leads to the woman being blamed by her parents, who at the same time feel guilty for causing what they do not want to accept in their daughter. For those women who may be forced to come out as a lesbian while they are seriously ill, encountering such reactions will be especially stressful.

4 Safer Sex

All sexually active women, particularly those whose partners are at risk or who are unsure of their partner's sexual background, need to know about ways of reducing the risk of contracting the virus which can lead to AIDS .

Apart from access to information, the degree of control women have in sexual relationships with men will seriously affect how able they are to reduce their risk of HIV infection. For instance, a man can choose to protect himself by wearing a condom, but a woman has to ask a man to agree to this.

Communication is vital to safe sex. It is important that you say what you want, and negotiate what you can do together. Many women will find this a difficult thing to do. We don't have a language for talking about sex that is easy to use. It's often hard to find words that are not too medical, vague or offensive – particularly as many are used in a derogatory way about women. Also, women are taught to be afraid and ashamed of sex. We often feel guilty if we talk about sex and what gives us pleasure. Some women may not feel able to talk about sex with their male partner, especially at the start of a sexual relationship – perhaps because they would feel too embarrassed or are afraid of how he would react. For instance, they may be afraid of being rejected by their partner or that he might leave them or, in some cases, become violent. There may be economic or cultural reasons why a woman may not feel that she has much say over what happens in bed. Within some marriages, for example, sex may almost be a bargain, part of what a husband expects of a wife in return for supporting her and any children they might have.

It's unrealistic and, to some extent, irresponsible to advise women to practise safer sex, without first acknowledging the problems and conflicts so many women face in taking charge of their sexuality. Women get raped and sexually abused. Women often have difficulty even getting their male partners to agree to use a condom – let alone abandon the idea that sex equals intercourse.

Beliefs about how women and men are expected to behave sexually also are important. Whilst for boys sexual experience is valued, this is not the case for girls. A girl who is 'prepared' for sex (e.g. by carrying condoms) is often perceived to be a 'loose' woman, on the look-out for sex. We don't talk about boys being slags if they 'sleep around', but if girls do this they risk their reputation. Similarly, a girl who suggests using a condom or mutual masturbation or other forms of non-penetrative sex also risks her reputation, as well as possibly losing her boyfriend. She may, for instance, be blamed for making the man feel sexually inadequate because she has gone beyond her expected role in taking the sexual initiative.

Clearly for many women, both young and old, the facts will not be enough. Knowing about how to prevent HIV infection is not the same as being able to put that knowledge into practice. For this reason, sex education should not just be about providing information. What is also needed are ways to help women feel more assertive and say what they expect and want from sex.

Equally, if more men had a different attitude to sex women would not have to ask their male partners to wear condoms or consider alternatives to penetration. What is also required, therefore, are ways to encourage men to consider the risks of sex and not leave the responsibility for the safety of sex up to women. Undoubtedly, this will not be easy. The majority of men have not had to think about the consequences of their sexual behaviour, for *themselves*, in any serious way before, while women have always had to.

Although there is no reason to believe that men are

incapable of making changes in their sexual behaviour,
many men will be reluctant to do so. The reasons for this are
complex and relate to the meanings attached to sex. As part
of the social construction of male sexuality, many men
come to believe that sex is both more important and more
uncontrollable for them than it is for women, that men and
not women should take the sexual initiative, and that what
counts as having sex is penetration of the vagina by the
penis. In addition to this, having sex, but more especially
having intercourse, is seen as a central aspect of being
masculine and male. One reason therefore why men, both
heterosexual *and* gay, may be unwilling to alter their sexual
behaviour in the light of AIDS is that such changes would
represent a threat to their identity. Another possible reason
is that they do not see safe sex as erotic, and assume they
won't enjoy it. While some men may be willing to agree that
satisfying sex need not imply intercourse, others will not.
For them safe sex may seem dull or uninteresting sex, a
poor substitute for the 'real thing', which would impose too
many restrictions on their sexual pleasure. Men who think
this have a lot to learn about sex, not least that defining sex
only as penetration is very limiting.

Whilst it may not be easy to change sexual habits, clearly
it is possible. Studies of gay men indicate that over the last
few years they have changed their sexual practices in the
light of AIDS. If gay men, many of whom are unfamiliar
with using condoms for contraceptive reasons, can change
then so too can heterosexual men.

Unlike gay men, many heterosexual men lack the motivation to change. They either don't see AIDS as affecting
them or, if they do, deny it because they are afraid that by
acknowledging their concerns they might be thought of as
gay or bisexual. But their homophobia could put them and
their sexual partners at risk. For instance, I've heard IV
drug users who regularly share equipment to inject drugs
proclaim – 'I'm not gay so how can I get AIDS!' And even if
many heterosexual men may not seem to be at risk from
AIDS, many heterosexual women *are* at risk from

unwanted pregnancies, cervical cancer, and other sexually transmitted diseases through unprotected intercourse. As far as women's health is concerned using a condom makes a great deal of sense.

Workshops on eroticising safe sex, and safe sex porn and erotica, are examples of attempts being made to change sexual attitudes and behaviour among men. In particular, they may enable them to realise that safer sex can be fun, exciting, and satisfying.

Apart from selling the idea of safer sex, using a condom will also have to be 'sold' to men through public advertisements on television and radio, in cinemas and in newspapers and magazines. The way some manufacturers have approached this is to associate wearing a condom with being macho. For example, the advertising slogan of a brand of condom called Jiffi was 'Real Men Come in a Jiffi'. In the United States slogans such as 'I like my Miller Lite and my condom tight' or 'Are you man enough for safe sex?' represent a similar attempt to appeal to a desire among men to prove themselves to be masculine. This may persuade some men to use condoms. It will not however challenge the fundamental association of masculinity and sexual performance, which is at the very root of women's sexual oppression.

Because of the different meanings attached to female sexuality, women are likely to need less convincing that safe sex can be both good for you *and* fun. Sexual surveys show that, generally speaking, women are more dissatisfied with their sex lives than are men and that, very often, their dissatisfaction is related to sex being defined primarily as intercourse. The fact that AIDS forces us to question many of the assumptions we hold about sex may, therefore, in some ways be regarded as positive.

This is not to ignore the fact that for some women AIDS has meant sexual difficulties. If they or their partner has AIDS, is antibody positive, or thinks they may be infected with the virus, anxieties about the consequences of having sex may lead to a loss of sexual desire. Some women may also be worried and fearful about sex because they are unsure about whether their partner may have had sex with someone else who might be at risk, and not told them. Such fears will be even greater for women whose partners expect and, in some cases, force them to have risky sex.

There are women who are busy going over their sexual histories trying to work out if anyone they slept with was 'at risk'. If you are worried about past sexual relationships you should carry out a 'risk-assessment'. The likelihood of your being infected will depend on a number of factors. When did the relationship take place and where? Was it with someone whose activities put them at risk for AIDS? What kind of sex did you have? If you had oral, anal, or vaginal intercourse did you use a condom? How often did you have sex with one another? For example, a woman who had unprotected vaginal intercourse regularly during 1987 with an IV drug user living in Edinburgh could well have been exposed to the virus and, in case she was infected, should take precautions to avoid giving the virus to anyone else. The same precautions would protect her against future infection if she wasn't infected already.

The HIV antibody test will tell you if you have been infected. However, because of the impact that a positive result can have on a person's life you should think carefully about taking the test and should only do so after proper counselling about what the test results mean. (For a fuller discussion see pages 2–4.)

How women feel about safer sex will depend on their attitudes towards sex. To what extent is sex an important part of their lives and how they see themselves? What does sex mean in their relationships? What kinds of sex do they enjoy most? How many different partners have they had over the past year? The difficulties women may have in making changes in their sexual behaviour are likely to depend on the answers to these and similar sorts of questions. For example, some women may experience difficulties in adapting to risk reduction guidelines because they feel frustrated at the thought of having to have fewer sexual partners. While this is seen as something that men are likely to experience, it is often assumed that women want to be monogamous. Not all women would agree. Equally, the assumption that sex isn't as important to women as it is to men may result in AIDS-related sexual difficulties and fears in women being ignored.

How can a woman reduce her risk of AIDS?

There are several ways in which you can reduce your risk of becoming infected with HIV and, possibly, developing AIDS. Basically speaking it is important that you have safe sex with men or women who may be at risk for HIV infection, their sexual partners, or with people who have AIDS, other HIV-related illness, or are antibody positive.

If you already have AIDS, are antibody positive, or think you might be infected with the virus, you should *always* follow risk reduction guidelines. Some people may feel that if they have already been infected with HIV they have nothing to lose by continuing to engage in unsafe sex. However, even though they may not have AIDS, they may be infectious to others and those persons may get AIDS. In addition to this, some doctors believe that repeated exposure to the virus may increase the likelihood of an infected person progressing to AIDS. By following risk reduction guidelines a person may therefore reduce the risk to themselves of getting AIDS, even though they are already infected with HIV.

The risk of acquiring any sexually transmitted disease rises with the number of different sexual partners you have. Similarly, with AIDS the more people you have sex with the more likely it is that at least one of them will be infected with the virus that causes it. This is especially true if you have sex with people whose behaviour puts them at risk. One way of reducing the risk of contracting the virus therefore is to be more selective about who you have sex with. (However, being monogamous is no protection against AIDS if your partner is already infected with HIV.) Know your sexual partner, his state of health, his lifestyle, and his sexual habits (past and present). Avoid having sex with men you know little or nothing about. Talk to any potential sexual partner and try to ascertain whether he is at risk, or has been in the past, before you make love. (Likewise make your own risk status known to him.) Ask him if you are the only sexual partner he has. Does he have sex with other men, even occasionally? (Remember a man may identify himself as heterosexual, but it's not what he *calls* himself that matters, it's what he *does*.) Does he ever inject drugs and share needles with other users? Is this something he used to do before he met you?

You should also negotiate with your partner what you can do *before* you start having sex. Don't leave it to the last minute. For instance, you might begin by asking 'How often have you tried safe sex?' or 'What brand of condoms do you like the best?' They may be relieved that you've raised the subject. Alternatively, they may interpret what you're saying as implying something negative about them. If he gives you a hard time and tries to make you feel guilty, for instance by asking 'Don't you trust me?', don't give way. You could tell him that you like him and that your reason for wanting to stick to safe sex has nothing to do with not finding him attractive. It's just that you make it a rule that if you decide to have intercourse to always use a condom. (You might also negotiate safe ways of being sexual that do not involve using a condom.) That way you can have fun as well as protecting *both* of you. If he still refuses to discuss it, or puts you down, you must ask yourself do you want a relationship with someone who doesn't respect your right to have the kind of sex you want?

If you don't feel able or don't know how to bring up the subject of safe sex with someone you've just met, start by finding out what he thinks about AIDS generally. One way you might introduce it into conversation is 'I read an article about AIDS the other day that disturbed me. I'd like to know what you think.'

One of the difficulties for women in doing this, apart from any embarrassment which they may feel, is that men may not answer their questions truthfully. When you are not sure if a man may be infected with HIV either don't have sex with him or follow risk reduction (safe sex) guidelines – unless you want to run the risk of becoming infected yourself. Don't be pressured into having sex because, for example, he says he won't love you any more if you don't, or alternatively, that he will love you forever if you do. He might just be saying that to get you to have sex with him. *Avoid using alcohol and drugs when you have sex.* They may impair your judgement, affecting decisions about who you have sex with and what kind of sex you have.

This will be more difficult for some women than others. Some women will be at risk of being beaten up or raped if they insist on safe sex. For many others being told to 'get rid of him' if, say, he refuses to use a condom will be neither practicable nor, in some cases, what a woman wants. One solution for women who are in this situation is to use other health concerns to persuade their partner to change. One woman told her husband that she had been told by her doctor that if she stayed on the pill she could develop thrombosis and die. Another woman told her lover that she couldn't use a diaphragm for birth control because she had a tipped uterus.

Some ways of having sex are more likely to transmit the virus than others. For transmission to occur, semen (or blood) containing HIV must enter a woman's body through her vagina, rectum, mouth or open cuts or sores on her skin. Researchers are not yet sure whether the virus can just pass through the moist mucous membranes which line the mouth, vagina and anus, or whether it gets directly into the bloodstream through tiny tears or abrasions. In men, a possible route of infection is through the moist entrance to the urethra (the small opening at the tip of the penis) In uncircumcised men it might also be possible for the virus to gain entry through the moist skin which is covered by the foreskin when the penis is not erect.

Sex that does not involve semen, blood or vaginal fluids coming into contact with the moist skin which lines your mouth, vagina, rectum or urethra, or open cuts or sores, is generally considered safe. Having said this, there is still some disagreement among AIDS researchers over what may or may not be safe sex. This is hardly surprising given that there is so much that is not yet known about HIV and how it is transmitted. In the light of this some prefer to use the term *safer* sex or risk reduction.

Only you can decide what is an acceptable amount of risk. Hopefully, the following guidelines, based on what is currently known about HIV transmission, will help you to make informed choices. Though it includes information of relevance to all women, this section is primarily aimed at women in heterosexual relationships. Information on safer sex for lesbians is contained in the previous chapter.

In each of the situations described below the practices are risky only when one or more people taking part are infected. You *don't* become infected simply by having certain kinds of sex.

Anal sex

Studies have shown that anal intercourse is the main way in which HIV is sexually transmitted among men. Women can also become infected with HIV through anal as well as vaginal intercourse.

The walls of the rectum are designed to absorb fluids readily and are very thin. They can easily be damaged during anal intercourse, allowing the virus to enter the bloodstream, carried either by semen or by blood from an injury to the penis. Even if there is no tissue damage, it may be possible for semen infected with HIV to get into the bloodstream during anal intercourse.

By far the safest solution is to avoid intercourse. However, if despite the risks you are having anal inter-course you should insist that your partner wears a condom.

Below is a list of different ways of having sex. Some of the
ways are described as safe sex. These are activities which
are believed to carry little or no risk of the virus being
passed from one person to another. Others are marked
possibly risky because they carry some risk of transmitting
the virus, although not as much risk as the types of sex
listed as high-risk.

Safe sex
- Massage.
- Hugging.
- Kissing.
- Hand and/or finger-to-genital contact if there are no cuts
  or open sores on your hands.
- Body-to-body rubbing.
- Sex toys, providing that they are not shared.
- Body kissing (away from the genital region).
- Mutual masturbation.
- Sharing sexual fantasies.
- Any sexual activities that do not involve the exchange of
  body fluids.

Possibly risky
- Oral sex (cunnilingus) by a man to a woman (or woman
  to woman), especially during her period. Using a latex
  barrier may reduce the risk.
- Vaginal intercourse with a condom.
- Anal intercourse with a condom.
- Oral sex by a woman to a man (fellatio).
- Semen, urine or faeces in the mouth, vagina or rectum.
- Fisting (hand in rectum or vagina) without protective
  gloves.
- Sharing sex toys used for penetration without cleaning
  or using condoms.
- Rimming (oral-anal contact).

High-risk
- Vaginal intercourse without a condom.
- Anal intercourse without a condom.
- Any type of blood contact (including menstrual blood).

Although it is not known how effective they are in real-life situations, studies have shown that condoms can prevent the transmission of HIV in the laboratory. For this reason most researchers believe that, when used properly, condoms reduce the risk of contracting HIV during vaginal and anal intercourse. (Do not go from the rectum to the vagina without changing condoms.)

Condoms reduce the risk of becoming infected with HIV; they do not make sex 'safe'. They have about a 10 per cent failure rate in preventing pregnancy, and the protection they provide against HIV infection could be lower since a woman can get pregnant only a few days each month but is at risk of HIV infection every time she has intercourse with an infected partner.

One reason for condom failure is people not using them properly. (The correct way to use condoms is described on page 96.) Sometimes the condom gets damaged, or else it is put on or taken off incorrectly. Another reason is the condom breaking. Only when the condom remains intact can the possibility of becoming infected with HIV be reduced.

Since condoms can fall off or tear during intercourse, it is safer for the man to withdraw his penis before he ejaculates. The major causes of condoms breaking are air inside the condom, not enough lubrucation, old or faulty condoms, or the use of oil-based lubricants.

Apart from helping to prevent the condom from ripping, the use of a lubricant during anal sex will also help to reduce friction and possible damage to the rectal walls. If you use a lubricant you should make sure it is a *water-based* lubricant, like KY Jelly or Duragel. You should not use Vaseline, or any oil-based lubricant, as they dissolve the rubber. Do not use saliva as a lubricant. It is not a very good lubricant and it may contain the virus if you or your partner are infected.

There is some evidence that nonoxynol-9, a chemical agent which is found in most spermicides and some lubricants, may afford some protection against HIV infection.

How to Use Condoms Correctly

- Open the package carefully so that you do not damage the condom.
- Hold the closed end of the condom between thumb and forefinger to squeeze out the air. Air bubbles can cause condoms to break. With plain end rubbers you need to pinch the end to create a space for the semen.
- Put a dab of water-based lubricant in the tip of the condom before putting the condom on. The lubricant helps keep the air out of the tip and will also increase sensation for the man.
- Unroll the condom so that it covers the entire length of the erect penis. Check that you are unrolling it the right way. When putting a condom on an uncircumcised penis, pull back the foreskin before rolling on the condom.
- Use a water-based lubricant on the outside of the condom before intercourse, preferably one containing nonoxynol-9. (Insufficient lubrication can cause condoms to tear or pull off.) Do not use oil-based lubricants or saliva.
- Sometimes, for example if the penis is getting soft, the condom may tend to slip or come off. Holding the base of the condom will stop it from slipping.
- After sex, the man should withdraw his penis before it becomes soft. One of you needs to make sure that the condom is held firmly around the base so that no sperm can be spilled.
- Throw the used condom away.
- Condoms should not be used more than once. Use a new condom *every* time you have sex.)

Studies have shown that under laboratory conditions nonoxynol-9 can kill the HIV virus. This does *not* mean that if you use a lubricant and/or a spermicide containing nonoxynol-9 you won't get AIDS. The body and the laboratory are very different environments and no one knows yet how effective nonoxynol-9 is against HIV during sex. Spermicides and lubricants should only be used as a backup to condoms, not by themselves.

Opinion differs on the amount of nonoxynol-9 which is needed to kill HIV in the test tube. Some researchers claim that nonoxynol-9 kills the HIV virus outside of cells at 0.05 per cent, but is ineffective against HIV inside cells until it reaches 2.5 per cent. Most spermicides at present contain between 1 per cent and 5 per cent. Foams contain the highest concentration of nonoxynol-9, up to 12 per cent. Foams are also more effective than gels at providing a chemical barrier, as they spread more evenly and cling better to the walls of the vagina.

Although it is not usual, some women are allergic to nonoxynol-9. If it irritates the skin it could make it easier for the virus to get into the bloodstream. You should therefore first test any product containing nonoxynol-9 on the side of your wrist before using it for sex. If you do get an allergic reaction try using a different brand. Nonoxynol-9 has been approved for vaginal and oral sex. It is unclear yet whether it can be safely used in the rectum.

Condoms come in different colours, flavours, textures and styles. They may be dry or lubricated, smooth or textured, straight or shaped, natural or brightly coloured. Some have a reservoir at the tip, others are plain ended. If you use this type make sure you leave a space at the end for the semen so it doesn't get forced up the sides. (Check there is no air in the tip of the condom which could cause it to break.) Buy some different brands and experiment to find out which is the right one for you both. Practise using condoms and learning (safely) what it feels like if the condom breaks. Lubricants, spermicides and condoms can be bought in most chemists.

Lubricated condoms – some are lubricated with nonoxynol-9 – do not break as easily as unlubricated ones. Another way of reducing the risk, and the worry, associated with the condom breaking is to use a *strong* condom. Condoms which carry a British Standards Institute kitemark have been tested for strength and reliability. More

important than thickness for strength is the age of the
condom and the way it is treated before and during sex.
Don't test condoms by blowing them up or stretching them.
Don't store condoms for a long time, or near heat, or in
strong sunlight. Don't use old condoms. Check the expiry
date on the packet. If it is past the 'use by' date, or hasn't
got one, don't use it.

If the condom does break, the man should slowly withdraw his penis. *Do not douche*, as this may create small
tears and increase the risk of infection. Consider instead
putting a large amount of spermicide containing 5 per cent
or more of nonoxynol-9 into the anus or vagina.

Other forms of anal sex, besides anal intercourse, can
also be dangerous. Putting vibrators or other sex toys into
the rectum could be risky as they could pass the virus from
one person to another if they are shared. 'Fisting,' inserting
the entire hand into the rectum and balling it into a fist, is
likely to cause tears in the walls of the rectum. This
increases the chance of contracting HIV should one have
anal intercourse afterwards. Fisting can also lead to a
number of other very serious, potentially fatal injuries and
infections, such as peritonitis. If, despite these risks, you do
this, you or your partner should always use a disposable
rubber glove. These are made of very thin rubber and can
prevent blood infected with HIV from coming into contact
with open cuts or skin rashes – like eczema – on your
hands. Similarly, if you have cuts or scratches on your
fingers wearing a disposable rubber glove will reduce the
risk of becoming infected with HIV during anal penetration
with fingers. Throw the glove away afterwards. Never go
from the anus to the vagina without changing gloves.
Disposable rubber gloves can be bought in most chemists.

Sex which involves faeces in the mouth, vagina or
rectum, or through cuts, could represent a risk as it may
contain blood. This includes oral-anal contact, also known
as analingus or 'rimming,' especially when there are cuts in
the mouth or gum disease. Faeces in the mouth or through
cuts may have caused a small number of transmissions.

Apart from the possibility of contracting HIV, oral contact with faeces may lead to a number of serious infectious diseases, such as hepatitis B. While it is safest to avoid these activities, using a barrier that prevents the exchange of fluids between the tongue and anus may reduce the risk of HIV transmission if you do have oral-anal sex. Dental dams, which are a thin piece of latex about the same thickness as a disposable rubber glove, can be used for this.

Vaginal intercourse

Vaginal intercourse also carries a high degree of risk for infection with HIV. HIV can be transmitted in semen entering the vagina. The virus might get into the bloodstream through ulcerations or erosions of the cervix or, possibly, through the vaginal walls. Though much thicker than the rectum, the walls of the vagina contain many blood vessels which become swollen with blood during sexual arousal. There may also be ulcers or tiny tears caused by friction during intercourse. Cuts or sores on a woman's genitals may also allow the virus to enter her bloodstream, carried either by semen or by blood from the man's penis. Because it can create small tears, douching before or after sex may also increase the risk of transmission. Such small tears or injuries will most likely not be noticed.

Many researchers believe that the risk of the virus being transmitted from a man to a woman during sexual intercourse is greater than the other way around. Studies both of gay men and female partners of men who inject drugs, for instance, suggest that it is the person *receiving* semen who is at greater risk of infection during intercourse. Nevertheless, sexual transmission of HIV from women to men can occur. The vaginal secretions of infected women may contain the virus, though it is thought that menstrual blood from women who have the virus probably holds a greater risk of infection. As with male-female transmission, the virus may be passed more easily from a woman to a man if there are cuts or abrasions on the penis, or a dry and inflamed urethra, which would allow the virus more direct access to the bloodstream.

One way of eliminating this risk is not to have intercourse. Because this demands the co-operation of men, this may be difficult to achieve in practice. It's no good a woman wanting to make love without having intercourse if the man she is having sex with won't agree.

If you do have intercourse, your male partner should always use a condom. Condoms cannot provide absolute assurance since they can come off or break, but most researchers believe that used properly they offer some degree of protection from HIV both to the woman and her male partner. Many studies have shown them to be effective in preventing other sexually transmitted diseases such as gonorrhoea, syphilis, and herpes.

Condoms should be used with spermicidal jelly or foam and a water-based lubricant containing nonoxynol-9. Since the condom may break, it is also safer for the man to withdraw before ejaculation. A further measure of protection is for the woman to use a diaphragm or cervical cap, with a spermicidal cream or gel containing nonoxynol-9. A diaphragm and cervical cap would protect the cervix and the uterus but not the vagina. By itself, therefore, a diaphragm is *not* sufficient protection against infection. But it may add to the safety of sex during a woman's period, when the walls of the uterus may be more receptive to infection. And, by blocking the blood flow from the uterus into the vagina, it may reduce the risk of infection to men having vaginal or oral sex with a woman who is infected.

Condoms are readily available, relatively inexpensive, and, with practice, are easy to use. (Family Planning Clinics provide condoms free.) They have no adverse side-effects and when used in conjunction with a spermicide are an effective means of birth control. Their serious disadvantage for women is that it is necessary to get men to agree to use them. (This may not always be the case. Testing has begun on an insertible condom for women, called Femshield.)

While this will not be a problem for all women, some men don't like condoms and may refuse to wear one; in some cases, some men may force their partners to engage in unprotected intercourse.

Men who refuse to practise safer sex may be putting both women and themselves at more risk. Why? The argument that 'it doesn't feel as good with a condom' is certainly not a good enough reason to put your own or someone else's life at risk. It's also not necessarily true. Condoms make sex safer; they can also make sex more exciting. Some men who climax too quickly find that wearing a condom can delay this and give them and their partner more satisfaction. For men who have difficulties maintaining an erection, a condom which fits tightly will tend to make erections harder and orgasms more intense. Condoms also cut down on friction, especially the lubricated kind. This can aid women who experience vaginal dryness and find intercourse uncomfortable.

Many women and men also find that by using condoms they are less worried about the various risks associated with intercourse and are therefore more relaxed and can enjoy sex more.

It's also important to remember that sexual intercourse is not essential to having satisfying sex. For many people having an orgasm by masturbation, whether you take it in turns to touch each other or do it simultaneously, is just as – if not more – enjoyable than intercourse. There is nothing wrong or abnormal about this. Even for those who think of 'real sex' as penetration, masturbation can be extremely pleasurable and it is very much safer than intercourse. Intercourse has rarely, if ever, been risk-free. HIV is one more reason to think about what part, if any, intercourse plays in your sex life.

Apart from the risk of infection with HIV, vaginal intercourse can result in pregnancy. As I have discussed earlier, pregnancy in women who are infected may lead to the virus being passed on to the foetus as well as, possibly, increasing the chances of their developing AIDS. If you or your

partner do things that put you at risk, or if either of you
have been diagnosed as having AIDS or being antibody
positive, then you should consider deferring pregnancy.
This is discussed in more detail in Chapter Two. While
alternative forms of birth control to the condom, such as
the pill or an IUD, may be effective in preventing pregnancy, they will not protect you against becoming
infected with HIV or other sexually transmitted diseases.
Therefore, you should *always* use a condom during
vaginal intercourse, irrespective of whether or not you are
already using some other method of contraception. There
is also a suggestion that semen can be immunosuppress-
ive for women. If this is the case, as well as protecting her
male partner, using a condom might help prevent women
who are sero-positive from progressing to AIDS or other
HIV-related illness.

Other forms of vaginal sex also carry a risk. Inserting
fingers or a hand into a woman's vagina – 'fisting' – may
cause bleeding. Wearing a surgical rubber glove, especially
if the person has cuts or scratches on their hand or fingers is
advisable, particularly during a woman's period. (You
should rinse the gloves before using them if they have been
treated with talc.) Rubber gloves also cause less friction
than bare hands and reduce the risk of tears or scratches.
Sharing sex toys such as vibrators that have come into
contact with semen, blood or vaginal fluids could also result
in the virus being transmitted from one person to another.
Protect sex toys that are shared by using a condom – use a
new condom for each person.

Apart from semen and blood you should also not allow
faeces to come into contact with your vagina (it may
contain blood). 'Water Sports' or 'golden showers' refers
to urinating on or in someone. There is no evidence so
far of HIV definitely being transmitted through urine.
However, as there may be blood cells which can transmit
the virus in urine, it is advisable not to let urine come
into contact with your vagina, rectum or mouth, or open
cuts.

Oral sex

Oral sex is where one partner stimulates the other's genitals with their mouth or tongue. When a man (or woman)
does this to a woman it is called cunnilingus. The term
used when a woman (or man) does this to a man is fellatio.

Whether the virus can be transmited orally, either by
oral-genital or oral-anal contact is not clear. Studies of gay
men suggest that it is difficult to transmit the virus orally.
However, until more is known about HIV and how it is
transmitted, oral sex should be considered to carry some
degree of risk. In fellatio this is because the virus could
pass from the man's semen into the woman's body. The
best way to avoid this is not having your partner ejaculate
in your mouth; although acids in the stomach probably
destroy the virus once it reaches the stomach, there may
be some risk of infection if there are cuts or sores in and
around your mouth and gums that would allow the virus
to enter your bloodstream. Apart from the risk from
infected semen, there is also the risk of being exposed to
blood infected with HIV if your partner has any small cuts
or abrasions on his penis. Withdrawing his penis before
ejaculation does not totally avoid the risk from semen,
since many men produce some secretion from the penis
prior to ejaculation. Men who perform fellatio for their
male partners obviously run the same risks as women who
do this. For men *receiving* fellatio, there is probably little or
no risk of infection. Although the virus has been isolated
in saliva, there is no evidence that it has caused transmission.

If you carry out oral sex for a man he should wear a
condom to reduce the risk of infection to you. Some
condoms taste awful because of their lubricants, others
have virtually no taste at all. For this reason, while lubricated condoms may be good for intercourse, you may
prefer to use an unlubricated condom for oral sex.

Since a condom can break, the man withdrawing before
he ejaculates is a further measure of protection. Although,

once again, the question of how much control women have within sexual relationships with men is a crucial one.

You could use a lubricant or spermicide containing non-oxynol-9, as well as a condom. If you do, you should first make sure that the spermicide or lubricant you are using doesn't irritate you or your partner's genitals, mouth, or (in the case of oral-anal sex) rectum.

Cunnilingus is thought to carry some degree of risk. Unless it contains blood there is little or no risk of HIV being transmitted through saliva. If there are no cuts or sores on a woman's genital area it is unlikely that she will become infected by her partner during oral sex. The main risk is to the man (or woman) doing this to her. The cervical and vaginal secretions of women infected with HIV may contain the virus. HIV is also likely to be present in a woman's menstrual blood. Therefore, if the person going down on a woman has bleeding gums, mouth ulcers, or any breaks in the skin in or around the mouth, the virus may be able to get into their bloodstream.

As the exchange of blood (and semen) is thought to carry a higher risk for infection with HIV than cervical and vaginal fluids, you should especially avoid having oral sex during a period. Using a thin rubber barrier that would prevent the exchange of fluids between the tongue and the vulva may reduce the risk of infection with HIV.

You could use dental dams for this (and for 'rimming'). These are disposable latex barriers which come in many sizes, colours, tastes, and thicknesses. You can obtain them from surgical and dental supply companies. (When you use dental dams, make sure to rinse them first. If they have been treated with talcum powder, this could irritate the vagina or rectum). Alternatively, you could cut a condom in half and use that. Condoms have the advantage of being easier to obtain and are usually thinner and more transparent than rubber dams. Unlubricated condoms taste better than lubricated ones. Using a water-based lubricant – preferably one containing nonoxynol-9 – between the latex barrier and the women's vulva will increase sensation.

Safe sex

So much of the talk about AIDS is about 'risky sex' that some people may feel afraid to do anything. While that is one solution, celibacy is unrealistic for most people. It is also unnecessary. AIDS doesn't mean no more sex. It means being aware of the many ways of having sex safely.

This doesn't mean no more fun either. Although you may enjoy intercourse, you certainly don't need to do this to have great sex. After all, many of us are in a sexual rut. Safer sex is an opportunity to improve our sex lives by exploring new ways of making love. Use your imagination. The possibilities for safer sex are practically endless. For example, below is a list of different ways of having sex. These are just some of the activities which are believed to carry little or no risk of the HIV virus being passed from one person to another.

- Hugging, massage, cuddling.
- Kissing.
  The only time when kissing might transmit the virus would be through French (deep or tongue) kissing where large amounts of saliva are exchanged. Even then, the risk is likely to be very low unless the saliva contains blood. While the virus has been found in saliva, there are no reports of people being infected through kissing.
- Body-to-body rubbing.
  Some people have orgasms by rubbing against each other's bodies. A woman may arouse herself and reach orgasm by rubbing her clitoris against her partner's thigh or arm. As long as there are no cuts or breaks in the skin this is safe. It is also considered safe if a man ejaculates onto a woman's body, providing that his semen does not come into contact with the anus or vulva and there are no cuts or breaks in the skin. Cover up any cuts or open sores on the body or hands with waterproof plasters.

- Penis rubbed between thighs or breasts.
- Touching your own genitals.
- Sucking a man's nipples.
- Masturbation.

  Masturbation, whether on your own or with someone else, is a good way of experiencing sexual pleasure. It is the way many women, even during intercourse, reach orgasm.

  'Mutual masturbation' is where both partners stimulate the other's genitals with their hands. Whether it is done mutually, or only involves one person touching another, the risk of transmitting HIV this way is very low. If you masturbate your male partner and have cuts, scratches, or sores on your fingers and hands, wearing surgical rubber gloves will reduce the risk of your coming into contact with semen containing the virus. Similarly, if a woman were menstruating and her partner had open sores or cuts on their hands there could be some risk of infection. Wearing disposable rubber gloves will reduce the risk of exposure to blood and cervical and vaginal fluids for men (and women) who stimulate a woman's genitals with their hands. In both cases, using a water-based lubricant containing nonoxynol-9 will increase sensation as well as adding a further layer of protection.

- Showering or bathing together.
- Sharing sexual fantasies.
- Touching your own genitals at the same time as your lover touches his or hers.
- Caressing and fondling each other.
- Using vibrators or other sex toys providing that they are not shared or are cleaned and dried thoroughly between each partner's use. Sex toys can be cleaned using household bleach diluted one part bleach to ten parts water. (Make sure the bleach solution is thoroughly washed off before use.)
- Sex talk.
- Touching a woman's breasts and nipples.

- Watching each other masturbate.
- Body kissing.

  Providing there are no breaks in the skin that could result in your being exposed to their blood, kissing your partner's body also carries little risk of acquiring HIV and can be extremely enjoyable. This includes kissing ears, neck, thighs, fingers, toes, hands, legs, etc.
- Touching a man's chest and nipples.
- Sucking on the nipples of a woman (providing she is not lactating or otherwise secreting).
- Anal penetration with fingers if there are no cuts or sores on your fingers or hands. Wearing a disposable rubber glove will reduce the risk of infection.
- Any activities that do not draw blood or involve body fluids which can transmit the virus coming into contact with body openings or breaks in the skin.

Safe sex is not just about AIDS. Safe sex won't get you pregnant. Safe sex won't transmit any sexually transmitted disease. Far from being a restrictive influence, safe sex may encourage new ways of making love which broaden our enjoyment of sex.

5 Living with AIDS

Most of what has been written about what it's like to have AIDS has been about gay men. There has been very little analysis of the experience of women who have AIDS, or are antibody positive.

This is a serious omission. The problems AIDS creates for women are not necessarily the same as those for men – gay or otherwise. For instance, women's access to health care, the support systems available to them, their ability to make changes in their sex life and their reactions to physical decline and disfigurement are likely to be different to men's. In addition there are specific problems which AIDS creates for women, such as in pregnancy.

It is important to discover how women feel, but this will not be easy. Most women with AIDS, or who are antibody positive, are reluctant to be interviewed. This is under-standable. AIDS is a stigmatising illness and they may have a lot to lose if it were discovered that they had HIV-related illness or were HIV positive. At present, very few women in this country have AIDS, which makes them all the more easily identifiable. (As of October 1988, 61 women had been diagnosed with the disease). In the United States, where over 6,000 women have been diagnosed with AIDS, the situation appears to be a little different. It seems that with greater numbers more women with AIDS or HIV infection are willing to discuss their experiences. This is one of the reasons I have used interviews with both British and American women. Another is that the British experience of

AIDS is a few years behind that of the United States. What many American women are experiencing today, more women in Britain are going to have to deal with. We therefore have the opportunity to learn from women living in the United States about issues that are going to increasingly affect us in future.

Finding out

Patty is 40 years old. She is an ex-heroin user. She lives in New York, where she has lived for most of her adult life. She originally came from Pennsylvania, where her parents still live. In the summer of 1985 Patty went back to visit them. She was not well. Her lover, with whom she had lived for eight years, had just died. Patty had also stopped using drugs and was going through withdrawal.

Patty stayed off drugs, but instead of feeling better she became worse. She was having fevers, had swollen glands and was bleeding vaginally practically non-stop. Though she had various tests no one could tell her what was wrong. Finally, in November, she was admitted to hospital with chronic pelvic pain. It was there that she was told that, in addition to having a large fibroid tumour in her uterus, she had ARC.

For some women a diagnosis of AIDS or ARC comes as a complete surprise. In Patty's case she was almost expecting it.

It really wasn't a shock. When he told me it was almost as if he was confirming something I already knew. By that time I had already got it into my mind that my lover had died of AIDS and that, among other things, he probably had pneumocystis pneumonia. He was very short of breath, and he had lost a lot of weight and he was having night sweats. I don't know for a fact that he died of AIDS, but I feel very certain.

Patty's lover was in his forties when he died. He had been diagnosed with endocarditis and liver problems. Like Patty, he was a heroin user. If he was infected, Patty could have contracted the HIV virus from him. They shared needles and didn't use a condom whenever they had intercourse.

Patty believes that there may be another explanation of how she came to get ARC. In 1979 she had a brief affair with a man who 'turned her on to drugs'. They had sex together without using a condom. She also shared needles with him, as well as with other people. Shortly after the affair ended Patty became ill. She was having night sweats, continually had swollen glands, and developed pneumonia and endo-carditis.

It's almost as if I could have infected John, if I was infected back in 1979. I mean maybe it's not true, maybe I only got this virus two or three years ago. But it's possible that I've had it for nine years already. That's something I'll never know, when I got it or how I got it. It could have been through a needle or it could have been through sexual contact. I gave up trying to figure all that out some time ago.

However much they are expecting it, for most people the news that they have AIDS or ARC is a shock. All kinds of questions may go through their mind: Can I start a family? Am I going to die? What's going to happen to my relation-ships? Will I ever be able to have sex again? This is how Patty felt:

I just thought that my life was over and the first thing I thought to myself was as soon as I get out of this hospital I'm going to get on the bus and go to New York and buy enough drugs to O.D. I'm going to kill myself.

Patty no longer thinks this way. She knows that a diagnosis of ARC or AIDS is not a death warrant. There is a life to live with ARC or AIDS, which for some people can be more fulfilling and meaningful than ones they were living beforehand.

Margaret is in her early thirties. She and her husband live in England. Four years ago she found out that she was antibody positive. She has never abused drugs and is not in any other risk group other than that her husband has haemophilia and unknowingly passed the virus on to her. Her initial reaction to finding out she was HIV positive was typical of many people:

> As soon as we sat in the doctor's office and he told us I thought, Oh God, what's hit us! I thought someone had hit me over the head with a hammer. I was just confused. I didn't know what to do. I didn't know what to expect.

Another common reaction is denial, which is often manifest by demands to be retested. Other reactions include anger and the feeling of being betrayed or cheated, anxiety and fear of losing control of bodily functions or mental faculties. But perhaps the most overwhelming reaction will be shock followed by depression and grief.

It is very difficult to take in information about the nature of AIDS, how HIV is transmitted, and what the possible implications of infection may be while being in a state of shock. Nevertheless, there are a number of issues which women who are antibody positive or have AIDS need to know about *soon* after diagnosis.

First, it is important they understand that they will most likely be infectious, even if they do not have any symptoms of infection themselves. Women who are aware of this may initially worry a great deal about the risk they pose to others. Very often, this is due to a misunderstanding of how HIV is transmitted. It is essential that women with AIDS, or who are antibody positive, have access to *accurate* information about how the virus is passed on and the steps that they can take to reduce the risk of this happening. Even then they may need reassurance. Margaret admits to being

If I have AIDS or am antibody positive what precautions should I take?

- Do not donate blood, plasma, body organs or other tissue. Men should not donate sperm.
- If you have sex with someone follow the risk reduction guidelines described in chapter 4 and, for lesbians, Chapter 3.
- Do not share needles or other equipment for injecting and mixing drugs.
- If you are considering pregnancy, or are already pregnant, you should consider carefully the possible risks to yourself and the risk of passing HIV to your child. Several of the organisations listed on p. 184 can put you in touch with people who are sensitive to the issues women face in coping with AIDS and pregnancy, including the decision of whether or not to breastfeed.
- Cover any cuts or grazes with a waterproof plaster.
- While studies do not show HIV transmission through the sharing of toothbrushes or razors, it is advisable to avoid sharing anything likely to be in contact with blood.
- Clean up any spilt blood or other body fluids immediately. Wash the surface down with one part household bleach diluted with ten parts of water.
- Dirty clothes, linen, towels, etc. should be washed in the hot wash cycle of an ordinary washing machine.
- Used sanitary towels and tampons should be flushed down the toilet, burnt or put into a sealed plastic bag and disposed of safely.

worried about giving the virus to others, despite the fact that she knows nothing she does is likely to put them at risk. 'I am terrified in case we give it to someone else. I know we couldn't really, but it's just the thought. It's silly to worry but I do.'

Patty also admits that when she was first diagnosed she was worried about giving the virus to others, despite the fact that she knew she was doing nothing to put them at risk.

I was in the hospital and my mother wanted to put her arms round me. I pulled away from her which was stupid because I knew I couldn't give her anything. But for some reason I just got this terrible feeling I don't want to give it to them and I pulled back and she just kind of stopped, you know. I think she was hurt by what I did, and confused, but it was just this fear, this irrational fear I had.

Some of the precautions that women who are antibody positive or have AIDS do need to take are listed on the opposite page.

In addition to information about how they can reduce the risk of passing the virus on to others, it is also important for women with AIDS or HIV infection to know how they can reduce their own chances of getting ill. The list on page 114 includes suggestions for improving – or maintaining – one's health. Some researchers believe that such measures may be helpful in the treatment of AIDS, as well as reducing the risk of those who are infected with HIV becoming ill. While there is no firm evidence for this, many people report feeling better as a result of making healthy changes in their diet and way of life.

Being infected with HIV does not necessarily mean you will get AIDS. But it is important that you know what the symptoms of AIDS and other HIV-related illnesses are so that you can monitor your own health and, if necessary, seek treatment quickly.

Apart from access to basic information, women should also have the opportunity to discuss how they feel. A woman who is diagnosed as having AIDS or as antibody positive has many issues which she will need to think about and come to terms with. Among these issues are treatment options, reactions by employers, family and friends, risk reduction, stigma and AIDS discrimination, feeling depressed and anxious, the physical effects of her condition, and dependency and finding support. In the following section some of these are discussed in more detail.

What should I do to protect my own health if I am antibody positive or have AIDS?

- If you can, eat a properly balanced diet and if you eat meat make sure it is well cooked.
- Try to cut down or cut out drugs which may damage your immune system.
- Try to reduce the amount of stress in your life.
- Get enough rest and sleep.
- Practise safer sex to avoid giving anyone else the virus, and you acquiring sexually transmitted diseases which may worsen your immune status.
- Wash your hands after handling pets and avoid contact with their wastes. Cat faeces expecially may harbour organisms which could cause serious illness in people with AIDS. If you can, either get a friend to clean the cat litter box or wear disposable rubber gloves.
- Try to avoid going to places where the sanitary conditions are poor and where there is a high risk of your developing infections. Normal standards of hygiene will be enough to protect you from household germs. Staying away from pubs, restaurants, cinemas, etc. is unnecessary.
- Do not accept any kind of vaccination unless your doctor knows that you are immune-deficient. While there is no risk from vaccines which contain killed virus, many vaccines have living – but altered – viruses which cause problems for someone with immune deficiency.

AIDS discrimination

Women with AIDS or HIV infection can face many problems. Some of these may be due to the way in which they are treated. AIDS is a severely stigmatising illness. There have been stories of nurses refusing to change bedpans, feed, wash, or even talk to someone in their care who has AIDS. In some cases people have been evicted from their homes or have lost their jobs once it became known that they were antibody positive or had AIDS. Insurance companies are unwilling to provide life cover. There are reports of people being abandoned by their friends, relatives and lovers, of children being excluded from schools, and of doctors refusing medical care.

At the hospital where she was first diagnosed with ARC, Patty received inferior treatment.

> The doctor told me plainly that he was afraid to operate on me now that they knew I was positive. They put me in isolation. Once something came into the room, it couldn't be taken back out except in a plastic bag. They brought in a big plastic bag for all the garbage and just left it there for seven days, never emptied it. The day I left there to go to another hospital it was really starting to smell. The whole room just smelled like a garbage dump. Nobody wanted to come in and see me. The nurses would just barely come in and throw the pillows at me, and when they did come in they got all dressed up in the garb, you know, caps and gowns and masks and gloves and boots, the whole works.

There is no need for hospital staff to wear gloves and masks, or caps and gowns just to go into an AIDS patient's room except in very special situations. Apart from being generally unnecessary, this can be upsetting for both the patient and their visitors. As Patty says:

> I couldn't bear to see my parents come to the hospital and have to go through putting on the caps and the gowns and the masks and the gloves in order to come to visit me. I didn't want to see them have to do that. I thought that would be a terrible, traumatic thing for them. So I told them that the doctor said I wasn't allowed to have any visitors.

Whatever form it takes, AIDS discrimination will be distressing for those who have HIV-related illness or are antibody positive. Some may respond angrily. Others, terrified of being found out, may become very anxious and withdrawn.

Isolation

Women with AIDS or HIV infection are often socially isolated. This may be because of the way people who are misinformed about AIDS and how HIV is transmitted react to them: with fear and avoidance. For many, such a response generates a feeling of being 'dirty' or 'unclean' and they may choose not to discuss their diagnosis with others for fear of how they will react.

The issue of who to tell is one that Patty has had to deal with. She decided to tell her parents the day she was diagnosed with ARC and has since told some of her friends in New York. She wants to be able to tell other people.

> I don't like being secretive. I went for so many years being secretive about drugs and I didn't like it. I don't want to have to be secretive about this; I want to be able to be open and honest about it.

While some people will decide to be very open about their diagnosis, others will decide they only want a few people to know. Apart from the hospital staff, only Margaret's close family know that both she and her husband are antibody positive. This decision not to tell friends or neighbours dramatically affected their social life.

> We stopped going out for months, just in case someone we met knew and they said anything. I didn't even think my mother should have known. I just didn't feel as if I trusted anyone to know, in case they mentioned it. What worries me about other people knowing is that they will treat me or my husband differently. I would have fears

of them not speaking, or just passing in the street, or not coming anywhere near the house.

There are other reasons, besides the fear that her friends will desert her, why a woman who is antibody positive or has ARC or AIDS may become socially withdrawn. She may have irrational fears about infecting others. She may also be concerned about the risk others present to her, in terms of catching germs and diseases. A woman's social life will also be affected by the physical effects of her diagnosis. Women with AIDS or other HIV-related illness may be too ill, or too easily tired, to be able to go out or socialise often.

Another reason why someone with AIDS may not mix socially is because they feel too upset or embarrassed about their physical appearance. Apart from weight loss, a person with AIDS may have disfiguring lesions on their face as well as on other parts of the body. The effect of having visible lesions in the case of a disease which is socially stigmatising should not be underestimated. Both chemotherapy and radiation therapy have been used in treating Kaposi's sarcoma lesions, which might otherwise identify someone as a person with AIDS. Unfortunately, those who undergo chemotherapy may also lose their hair. The impact of feeling unattractive on a person's self-esteem will vary with the individual. However, given that – far more than men – women are frequently judged in terms of how they look, such changes may be particularly stressful for women (although Kaposi's sarcoma is far less common among women than men.)

Whatever the reasons for social isolation, it is important that women who are antibody positive or have AIDS have someone to talk to. Talking can be a way of coping with the stress of diagnosis. Often it is practical problems which a woman feels she needs to discuss, as well as her fears and anxieties. A lover, friend or relative may be able to provide this. Alternatively, it may be helpful to join a support group. Support groups can provide the opportunity to learn from the experiences of others in a similar situation to yourself. They can also make you feel less alone. Meeting someone who is going through a similar experience to herself is something Margaret feels she would like to do.

> I feel very isolated and alone knowing that I don't know anyone in the same boat as me. They probably couldn't tell me anything I didn't already know, but I think it would just be nice to meet someone like me, because I would know what they'd be going through. I know there must be other women, but as far as I'm concerned I'm the only one. I just feel dead lonely.

Another advantage in joining a support group for women in a similar situation to oneself is that it offers the opportunity of meeting others without the fear of being rejected or ostracised.

Kristen is a black woman with AIDS. She got it, she says, through 'sleeping around' with different men. She lives in Los Angeles, and does voluntary work for an AIDS organisation there. She first became ill in 1983, when she was diagnosed with meningitis, Barr Epstein virus and cytomegalovirus. The doctors told her she would gradually get better. This turned out not to be the case. In 1985 Kristen was diagnosed with ARC. The following year, after the development of oesphagitus, she was told she had AIDS.

For Kristen, having a group she could turn to for support and help when she needed it has meant a great deal.

> Many people have asked me what my experience has been being black, being a woman with AIDS, being a heterosexual with AIDS, and they assume it was very lonely and very difficult and I have to say that, thank God, it was none of those things. I was fortunate inasmuch as when I realised I had AIDS I went straight to AIDS Project/LA, and they were wonderful. They supported me through a very, very rough period in my life, and with their support I pulled through beautifully.

Many of the support services currently available arose out of gay men's health concerns. Given the history of the AIDS epidemic it is hardly surprising that the focus of many support services is on gay men – however, this can exacerbate the sense of isolation many women feel. A woman may find that she is the only woman in a support group of all men. Also, many women feel uncomfortable discussing their sexual concerns in support groups with men.

When Patty first went along to Gay Men's Health Crisis in New York she was the only woman in her support group.

In the beginning it was very difficult for me to go there but there was nowhere else to go. All I knew was that this was a group of people who were helping people with AIDS and people with ARC, and that they had a lot of information and that they were offering a lot of services. So I said, I'm just going to have to take a deep breath and forget I'm the only woman here.

That was almost three years ago. Patty still takes part in a lot of the social activities run by Gay Men's Health Crisis. She also now belongs to one of the women's support groups that have been formed in New York.

Few support groups for women with AIDS or who are antibody positive exist in Britain at present, although many AIDS organisations do offer advice and support to women. In the London area, Positively Women acts as a support group for women with AIDS or HIV. The Terrence Higgins Trust can also put you in touch with other women in the same position as yourself or arrange for someone to visit you. Both these and other organisations offering help are listed on pages 184–94.

Anxiety

Most people feel shocked and disorientated when they discover they have AIDS or are infected with the virus

which causes it. They may refuse to accept the diagnosis
and become angry. Alternatively, they may react by
blaming themselves and feel depressed. Almost everyone
feels anxious and scared.

Anxiety is something we all experience at different times
in our lives. In this context, however, the anxiety felt is
likely to be far more severe and longer-lasting. A diagnosis
of AIDS is very frightening. It is, after all, a fatal disease for
which there is currently no known cure.

Knowing that she may develop AIDS is something Margaret feels anxious about. Whereas she rarely worried
about her health before being told she was HIV positive,
she now has to confront the possibility that both she and
her husband could become ill or even die.

> I worry about the future. Well, I've always been scared of
> dying anyway, always. When I lie there and I think my
> life could be cut short ... I'm terrified if anything
> happens to me. For instance, I'm scared now if I get a
> cold, I make sure I get it seen to straight away. I'm always
> at the doctor's. I worry about my husband as well. If he's
> not well I think has he got it? If something happened
> through haemophilia I could come to terms with that: it's
> dying of AIDS I worry about. That's very upsetting. I cry
> about that a lot.

The fact that AIDS occurs primarily in young adults
makes the prospect of death even more difficult to accept.
For many, however, the fear of death is not as great as the
fear of dying a slow and painful death, isolated from people
they know and care about.

Being rejected by family and friends is something that
women with AIDS and HIV infection are likely to be afraid
of. In addition, those already in a relationship may worry
about how their lover will cope with the diagnosis and the
issues it raises. In particular, they may be anxious about
how the sexual implications will affect their relationship,
and whether their lover will leave them for someone else.

Those who work may also be frightened that they will lose their job if their employer finds out about their condition.

There is still a great deal that is not known or understood about AIDS. In view of this it is easy to see how women who have the disease, or have been diagnosed as seropositive, may feel anxious for other reasons. For those with AIDS there is the uncertainty about how the disease will progress, the risks they pose to others, the effects of medical treatment and the possibility of a cure being developed. For those who have other HIV-related illness, or who are antibody positive, there is the uncertainty of whether they will go on to develop AIDS.

For many people with ARC or who are antibody positive, fear of AIDS becomes a constant source of anxiety. They may be able to think of little else but the prospect of developing AIDS and what the consequences of this would be. Often this means going over and over the same thoughts. For instance, they may be worried that perhaps they have given the virus to someone else already. Or, they may be consumed by thoughts of death and dying and watch themselves daily for symptoms of AIDS. In some cases the anxiety produced by such thoughts is so great that this develops into an obsession. The person feels compelled to check their body for signs of illness and may spend many hours each day doing so. In this context, for all of the tragedy, bitterness and anger that a diagnosis of AIDS can bring to the person who has HIV-related illness or is antibody positive, it may also be a kind of relief from the terrible uncertainty of not knowing whether they will develop the disease.

Knowing she has ARC has not, so far, caused Patty to become anxious, though, inevitably, she thinks about whether she will ever develop AIDS.

I do think about it a lot, maybe almost every day, and I just say, 'Well that's never going to happen, I'm never going to get full-blown AIDS. I'm going to take care of myself. I'm just not going to let it happen.' But always there is this thing in the back of your mind.

Unfortunately, many of the symptoms of anxiety and worry – sweating, feeling feverish, diarrhoea, weight loss, fatigue – are similar to those of AIDS. A woman who is worried about her condition may therefore mistake the symptoms of stress or a mild infection for signs that she is developing AIDS. This may make her feel even more anxious, causing a worsening of her symptoms, which further confirms her belief that she may have the disease. It is important, for this reason, that the symptoms of anxiety are explained to women with ARC or who are antibody positive soon after diagnosis.

Reading about AIDS in the newspaper or seeing something about it on the television can also be a source of distress and worry. One solution is to avoid the frequently inaccurate and gloomy coverage of AIDS in the media. Margaret no longer watches the news or reads a Sunday newspaper. 'I get upset if I read things in the newspaper or see something about AIDS on the television. I have a good cry. I don't believe everything I read, but it still upsets me.'

Depression

Four years after being diagnosed as antibody positive Margaret remains in good health. She keeps fit and shows no sign of developing AIDS or other HIV-related illness. Despite this, and the fact that she says she has come to terms with her condition, she frequently gets depressed.

I get depressed an awful lot. I've been depressed before, but not like this. I'll always find something on the subject to depress me. Like if I read a tiny clip in the paper I'll make a big scene over it. It's mostly at night, when I'm lying in bed. I haven't slept for about five or six nights now but I don't know why. I'm also getting really bad headaches but I don't know if it's tension or depression or what. I think it's because I'm tired and I get upset.

This is both a common and an understandable reaction. Most people become depressed when they find out that they have AIDS or are antibody positive. AIDS makes them feel that they no longer have any control over their lives. Their sense of helplessness is exacerbated by the fact that not only is AIDS incurable, it also tends to run an unpredictable course. Some people die quickly, whereas others may be in and out of treatment for several years, with periods of relatively good health interspersed between bouts of illness. The process of medical observation and treatment immediately following diagnosis of AIDS, which inevitably disrupts a person's normal routines, can also contribute to a feeling of loss of personal control and identity. Similarly, those who have ARC or are antibody positive may feel powerless to do anything to prevent themselves from going on to develop AIDS.

Feeling trapped and unable to do anything to change the situation, some women may become extremely despondent and lose interest in life. Activities which they previously found interesting and enjoyable start to become a chore, and they may stop going out or doing things they used to enjoy. There may be other reasons, besides feeling helpless, why someone with AIDS becomes depressed. AIDS is a physically debilitating and disfiguring disease. Many people with AIDS, especially in the latter stages of the disease, are weak and become increasingly dependent on others to look after them. They may also be in a great deal of pain and discomfort. Because of these physical limitations, a woman with AIDS may become isolated socially. Whether it is for this reason, or because of fears of how others will react, social isolation is another source of depression.

Women with AIDS or HIV who are depressed need to be encouraged to mix socially. As Margaret says, 'Lately I've been trying to get out more often to try and take my mind off things, because I think there's nothing worse than just sitting thinking.'

The preoccupation with illness and death which some women experience also makes it important to plan activities which are enjoyable. Establishing routines may also afford some distraction from anxious or depressing thoughts.

Apart from consistently feeling very low – that 'nothing's any fun any more' - someone who is depressed is likely to experience a number of other changes. They may find it difficult to concentrate, feel unable to cope even with simple tasks, lack motivation to do things, have problems sleeping, lose their appetite, and have no interest in sex.

They may also feel extremely guilty and blame themselves for all sorts of things, including their condition. Such reactions are most likely to occur when someone has become infected with HIV through activities which are not socially approved of. In women this usually means through IV drug use or certain forms of sexual activity, in particular where a woman is having sex with a number of different partners. The media portrayal of prostitutes and IV drug users (as well as of gay men) as somehow being to blame for the 'spread' of AIDS encourages feelings of self-recrimination and blame. While not all women will accept such definitions, those who do may experience a marked drop in self-esteem. They may also feel angry with themselves for 'causing' their condition. Patty went through a period of feeling this way.

> In the beginning I blamed myself; I said, 'I got what I deserved' but that was in the beginning. Now I don't look at it that way. I realise now that although I was using drugs I was a victim. It wasn't something that I really wanted to be doing. It was something that I was more or less pressured into doing because I was just at the end of my ropes, and I just couldn't deal with life anymore and I wanted to die.

The reactions of others to a diagnosis of AIDS or HIV infection can also have an important effect on a woman's self-esteem. A woman may feel like a 'social leper' as a result of being rejected by friends, lovers, family members or work colleagues. Changes in her physical appearance due to AIDS or other HIV-related illness can also contribute to a loss of self-esteem.

Given the nature of the disease, and the social and financial difficulties that women with AIDS and HIV infection often have to face, suicidal feelings may also occur. It may seem that the future is so bleak that life is simply not worth living any more.

Yet despite all the pain and the suffering that a diagnosis of AIDS or other HIV-related illness can bring, it's important to recognise that there can be good as well as bad times. Some people say that their diagnosis has given them greater self-knowledge and brought them closer to friends and family. Patty says:

> There is life after AIDS, after ARC, and life can be wonderful. I feel that, as bad as this disease is, for me it's been salvation. It's saved me from the terrible life I was having. I'm much happier now than I ever was before, and I'm a lot more confident and I like myself a lot more. So, for me, a lot of good has come out of this and I think you'll find a lot of other people with ARC and AIDS who will say the same thing.

Some researchers believe that relaxation and meditation techniques may help to overcome the sense of hopelessness which often signals rapid physical decline in many people diagnosed as having a terminal illness. The 'Simonton method', where a person visualises from a deep state of relaxation that their white blood cells are destroying the virus, is one such technique. Teaching relaxation and imagery techniques can also be useful in the management of anxiety.

As part of her efforts to stay healthy Patty practises visualisations.

> I imagine all these little work crews all through my bloodstream and they're all working on the virus, and then they shovel it into a truck and then the truck carries it to

my kidneys and then when I go to the bathroom it all comes out and is flushed away.

Another approach to dealing with AIDS and other HIV-related illness, which has clearly helped many people, is to develop a healthier lifestyle, for instance by making improvements in diet, exercising regularly, lessening stress and cutting out or cutting down on alcohol, cigarettes and other drugs that are known to damage health. Patty has stopped drinking and no longer uses drugs. She eats more healthily, goes to relaxation therapy and is trying to give up smoking. Doing all these things, she believes, helps to protect her immune system and reduces her chances of becoming ill.

Margaret takes regular exercise. She goes to keep-fit, swims regularly and enjoys going for long walks. She also takes care of herself in other ways:

> I don't drink a lot now because I know that lowers your immune system. I eat well. Of course I'm very conscious about my weight now in case I lose weight. I don't smoke. I keep myself wrapped up in winter. For instance, when I come out of the baths I make sure that I'm extra dry and my hair is dry because I don't want to get a cold.

Although there is no substantive evidence that any of these regimes can prevent or otherwise alter the course of AIDS, some researchers suspect that they may play a part in restricting the development of the disease. Certainly, they can do no harm and will increase the feeling of being in control of one's life and responsible, to a large extent, for one's own health. However, while these measures can give a sense of hope, many people find it difficult to make major changes in their lifestyle – such as stopping smoking or drinking. It's important to recognise this and also that change is a gradual process which takes time. Otherwise the danger is that people will set themselves unrealistic goals and feel that they've failed in their attempts to improve their own health if they find they can't change.

Sexuality

Sex may be a particularly emotive subject for women who are antibody positive or have AIDS, especially if they contracted the virus this way. Some women may feel sexually 'dirty' or unloved. Others may think that because they have AIDS, or are infected with HIV, they can't have sex any more. This is not the case. You can have sex providing that you make love in ways that do not transmit the virus.

Always have safe sex if you have AIDS or other HIV-related illness, or are sero-positive. Even if you have no symptoms, you will most likely be infectious and could give the virus to someone else who might become ill and die. You could also possibly reinfect yourself, which might possibly increase your own chances of going on to develop AIDS.

Patty has not had sex with anyone since she was diagnosed with ARC in November 1985. She says that this is because she hasn't met anyone she wants to have sex with. But she also recognises that having the virus has made her stop and think a lot more about it.

> I would be afraid of giving them the virus, even though I know all of the safe sex practices and I would certainly insist on using them. But I would still worry about giving the virus to someone else.

A woman who is antibody positive or has AIDS may need help and support in telling her sexual partner, or an ex-partner. Patty is aware that, if she did meet someone, this would be a difficult task. Nevertheless, she says she wouldn't have sex with anyone without first telling them she had ARC.

If I were going to have sex with someone I would want to
be able to trust them enough that I could tell them that I
have the virus and they could accept that. If they couldn't
accept that and go along with having safe sex then that's
not the person that I'd want to have sex with anyway. It's
not going to be easy. It's going to be really, really hard. I
can imagine going out on a date and saying 'tonight is
going to be the night that I tell him,' and then tonight is
not the night that I tell him. I know it is going to be hard
but I think that when the time does come I will have the
confidence to be able to tell someone.

Following risk-reduction guidelines may mean making
some changes in sexual habits. This may be difficult or
upsetting for some women. Certainly this applies to Margaret. Even though she feels that in many ways knowing
they are antibody positive has brought her and her
husband closer together, Margaret finds the recommendations have affected their lovemaking. She and her
husband also have sex less often.

When you are in the middle of it, it's still in your mind.
You can't enjoy it as much for that reason. I still very
much want to make love with my husband but the virus
is always on my mind. I have a good cry before sometimes, or afterwards. I can still enjoy myself, very much,
but it's restrictive, especially oral sex. I don't really kiss
my husband on the lips all that often any more. That's
difficult because I love smoochy kisses and he won't give
me one. It's just a peck usually. He's being more cautious
than me.

   I think it's been more difficult for him, definitely,
because if he'd known earlier, he'd have had it
chopped off. That's what he's always said. If he'd have
known he'd never have made love to me in the first
place. That's what he's upset about, the fact that he's
passed it on to me and that he didn't know. He feels so
guilty.

There are other worries about transmission specific to women. Anxiety about becoming pregnant is something which, to varying degrees, many women experience when they have sexual intercourse. This is especially true for Margaret. Like other women who are antibody positive or whose partners are, she has been advised not to have children on the grounds that she might pass the virus on to the child and, also, possibly increase her own chances of developing AIDS.

While some women may not, Margaret has found this very difficult to come to terms with. This is understandable. Women are expected to want children. Indeed, there are strong social pressures on women to see motherhood as a central aspect of their lives and their self-identity. Nevertheless Margaret has, reluctantly, accepted the advice she has been given and, as she says, is anxious to avoid pregnancy. 'I worry in case anything happens. If I ever became pregnant, what would I do? That's the biggest fear. I'm on the pill, as well as using the sheath.'

Women who have AIDS or are antibody positive and have children may have other worries. When a woman becomes ill with AIDS or other HIV-related illness, her traditional role within the family, especially as care-giver to a child or to other adults, may be seriously affected. She has to deal with a life-threatening illness, and she also has to deal with the impact on her family. A major issue for some women, especially if they are a single parent, is what will happen to my children if I become ill or die? They may also fear infecting their children, losing custody or seeing them ostracised as a result of their condition. In addition to the anxiety which such fears can provoke, some women may also feel guilty and ashamed: a failure as a mother. Women in this situation are likely to require services that often do not exist, such as help in dealing with their feelings and, if they do become ill, with planning for the future care of their children. It is essential that in future services be developed to encompass these needs.

6 Caring for people with AIDS

While women do get AIDS themselves, it is as carers of people with AIDS that the disease has, so far, had its biggest impact on women's lives. This is because those who do most of the caring for the sick, both within the home and outside it, are women.

Caring is an activity which is seen as natural for women. This is why occupations such as nursing, looking after the elderly and work with young children are generally thought of as 'women's work'. The assumption is that women have a natural aptitude for such work that most men lack. In some situations it is also regarded as their *duty* to care. As a wife and mother a woman is expected to care for her children, her husband, her husband's parents and her own parents (should they become ill or infirm), and, frequently, her grandchildren, if she has any. Such beliefs can produce feelings of guilt in women who, for whatever reasons, do not provide that care (working women, women with infirmities, etc.). In other situations women are often put in the position where they feel they have no choice but to stay at home caring for children or infirm family members, even when they would prefer to work outside the home and, often, need to for financial reasons. This is a real problem especially for women who don't have access to 'community care' programmes such as day care, etc.

This chapter looks at what it means to care for someone with AIDS, the dilemmas which caring poses for women, and the practical issues that can arise.

The experience of care

Finding out that someone you know has AIDS is likely to come as a tremendous shock. In many cases the shock of diagnosis is made worse by the fact that the person with AIDS has not previously said that they are gay or bisexual, or that they inject drugs.

Richard is in his early thirties, gay, and has AIDS. Though he decided not to tell his father he was gay his mother, Maggie, had known for a long time. She also knew when her son was diagnosed as antibody positive and worried when he started to lose weight and became progressively more and more exhausted. In the summer of 1986, her worst fears were confirmed. Richard developed pneumocystis and was taken into hospital. It was there that he told his mother that he had AIDS.

> Although you think you've prepared yourself, nothing prepares you for it. It was a *terrible* shock. Of course it was even more difficult for my husband because he'd never been actually appraised of the fact that Richard was even gay.

Apart from the initial experience of shock upon learning that a friend or relative has AIDS, most people will suffer from the same feelings of helplessness, very similar to those the person with AIDS is likely to be experiencing. They will feel considerable sorrow at the thought, not just of them dying, but also of the pain and suffering which they may have to endure.

Joyce Brink is fifty-five, married, and lives in Torrance, California. She and her husband originate from the Midwest, but have spent most of their lives in California.

Joyce worked as a secretary for many years. She is also the mother of three children.

Bill was her youngest son. Both Joyce and her husband had known Bill was gay since he was in high school. They also knew, in 1983, that Bill's lover had died of AIDS. For the next two years Bill remained healthy. Then, in the summer of 1985, he started to feel unwell. He lost weight, was often tired and had one bad cold after another. In December he started having diarrhoea and vomiting. Bill had planned to go away with his parents on holiday, but decided against it. When they returned three weeks after, he had lost twenty-five pounds in weight. Also, there were purplish spots on his right shoulder and on the end of his nose. The spots turned out to be Kaposi's sarcoma lesions and Bill was diagnosed as having AIDS.

This is how Joyce felt:

> I felt terrible, like the whole world had come to an end. All I could think of was how do we fight it, what are we going to do.

Depending on how the disease was contracted, some women may also be very angry. Many men, for instance, don't tell their wives or girlfriends when they have had sex with someone else, especially if it is another man. However they react, this will have an important bearing on their ability and willingness to care.

A labour of love

Caring is not just an activity, a form of work, it is also a set of feelings. When we talk about caring for someone we usually mean that we feel loving towards them and are concerned about their welfare. Caring, in this sense, is something many women want to, and expect to, provide, especially within the family.

Maggie feels this way about her son. She wants to care for

him and, although she knows this will get more difficult as his condition worsens, would find it dreadful not to be able to.

> I think that would be the worst thing that could happen, if I couldn't physically do it, that would be terrible for me. I don't look forward to it. It fills me with fear because you don't know how you're going to cope and you don't know what you'll have to cope with either. But not being able to do anything about it would be devastating.

Joyce also felt this way about her son:

> I had to be there. There was no other place for me. I *couldn't* go to work. It was so important for me to be there with him. He wasn't a burden. I didn't look at it that way.

In March 1986, Bill went into hospital for the first time. He had been steadily losing weight and was put onto IV fluids. Bill improved and, after a week, left the hospital. In April he was readmitted. This time as well as weight loss, he was having problems with breathing. Within twenty-four hours of admission one of his lungs collapsed.

Bill was unhappy in the hospital. He was in isolation and the care staff didn't look after him well. They would leave his food outside his door and didn't clean his room. Eventually Joyce and her husband decided to take Bill home, and arranged for home-health care.

After Bill came out of hospital Joyce left her part-time job to look after him. Bill was weak and frail as a result of pneumocystis and the diarrhoea. He was in bed and on IV fluids. With the help of the home-health nurses who visited him, Joyce quickly learnt how to operate Bill's IV, which she had to change three times a day.

Joyce didn't find the extra work involved in caring for Bill difficult. In her case it was the mental strain, the constant pressure of worrying about her son's health, which left her feeling tired and exhausted.

It didn't seem like it was the extra work, it was just the stress and strain of seeing him debilitated right in front of me and there was nothing I could do to stop it. No matter what I did or how hard I worked at getting the IV fluids into him, or helping him keep clean, or giving him food and nourishment, or whatever I could do, I was fighting a losing battle.

Those providing support and friendship to people with AIDS are in an unpredictable situation. Some people who have AIDS die suddenly, others may be in and out of treatment for several years. The uncertainty of knowing how the illness will progress can cause a great deal of stress, both for people with AIDS and for those caring for them at home. There is also the worry for Maggie that she may put her son at risk by passing on germs and diseases.

I had a bad cold so I decided although I was going to see him I wouldn't, because I was at the infectious stage and it's silly to court trouble. He's living an ordinary life and obviously he's going to come up against ordinary germs, but I wouldn't push him into any infectious situation.

In addition, those providing care share the difficulty of knowing how best to respond to someone whose mood is likely to fluctuate between hope and despair.
Joyce describes it as like being on a roller-coaster:

Bill would pick up and he'd start to gain weight. He'd start to feel better and be able to be up and around the house. Then all of a sudden, a few days later, he'd start with the vomiting and the diarrhoea and he would just go right back downhill. Then you have to put on the boxing gloves again and go on battling. I don't know where the energy comes from, you just suddenly find it, you have to call on inner resources to be able to cope with it. You just have to be strong because you have to be strong for him.

Joyce never lost hope. As she says, 'it's very important to encourage people to be hopeful, there *is* hope until hope is gone'.

When her son first came out of hospital Maggie looked after him for a month. He was not bedridden, but he was very weak and frail as a result of the pneumocystis and the side-effects of the drugs used in treating it. The extra work involved in caring for him, and since, Maggie has not found difficult. 'After all, between looking after two and looking after three is not a lot of difference really.' In her case the stresses and strains of caring are associated with the emotional aspects of providing care.

When you're actually coping with the worst parts of it, it's as if you've got some sort of power inside of you that keeps you going, keeps you putting on your make-up and making sure that you're looking good when you see them and, when you go to the hospital, that you're not down-hearted. But then, afterwards, you get very tired, terribly tired and for no good reason it seems. You just feel dreadfully tired.

One of the hardest things Joyce had to cope with was Bill's negative reaction towards her. Like many people with AIDS, Bill went through a stage of not wanting to see anyone. He became withdrawn and would often take out his feelings of anger and frustration on his mother.

It was terrible. I loved him so much I wanted to do everything I could, yet I felt like I was being completely rejected. I'd go in to say something or to check on him and he'd say 'What do you want'; he'd be very abrupt and hateful with me. I was being told, 'Go away mother I don't need you, get away from me, leave me alone'.

Because we feel it's safe to do so, people who love us are often the ones we direct our anger and frustration at. Part of Bill's reaction was also due to his feeling worried about his mother, and guilty at possibly being a burden to her.

Before he died Joyce and Bill were able to talk this through. Once she had convinced him that he was not a burden and that she wanted to be there Bill's behaviour changed. In fact Joyce says that one of the good things to come out of Bill's illness was that it brought him and his family closer together.

For other women there may be different stresses. Maggie is conscious of wanting to be supportive without being over-protective.

The stresses I find are not knowing what's going on inside him and knowing how far to push and how far not to push. For instance I would like to be much more demonstrative, but I hesitate. I suppose I'm looking for reassurance from him. I have no fear of Richard, but because I am so anxious about him I want to smother him and you can't do that. You see everything you do is two-edged in a way. You don't want to remind him that he's ill, and you don't want him to think that you're being crass. So you're walking a tightrope really.

Although Maggie does not, many women caring for someone within the home feel isolated and cut off from the outside world. This is likely to be particularly true of women who receive little or no support as carers. The decision whether or not to tell others will therefore be important in terms of how women caring for people with AIDS experience their caring role.

In Maggie's case, she felt that she had to tell many of her friends. This was partly because she didn't want them to think she was putting them at risk, especially those who had young children. 'A lot of them knew Richard was gay and, although they hadn't said it, when he got ill I know a lot of them suspected he had AIDS.'

Her decision was also based on how she thought she would be able to cope with the situation.

I felt totally selfish about it. I thought this is my situation
and I've got to cope with it the best way I can, and if I lose
friends well I've just got to lose them. In fact, I've had a
lot of support from my friends, they have been wonder-
ful about it. Mind you I haven't told everybody, I've been
selective. Some people are just bigotted and you don't
tell them.

AIDS-related discrimination can also affect people who
care for people with AIDS. Joyce admits that she did feel
isolated after Bill was diagnosed with AIDS.

In the very beginning I did, because I didn't know how
people were going to respond as far as even my own
family I wasn't too sure. I knew my sister would be
supportive, and my daughter and my elder son. I knew
they would be supportive, but I really wasn't sure about
neighbours or friends.

In fact, Joyce received a lot of help and support from the
friends she did confide in.

Friends would call round and ask is there anything you
want or that we can do? For example, the women from
my church called and they said can we come over and
clean the house for you, can we do your washing and
ironing? I just said everything's fine, you know, thanks
very much. A few days later one of them called back and
she said 'Joyce we're not going to wait for you to tell us
what to do, we've decided. We've had a meeting and
every Tuesday and Thursday night someone will be
there with dinner for you' and from the end of April until
Bill died in August every Tuesday and Thursday they
did.

Although Joyce feels fortunate in her friends, and has
been relieved and comforted by the sympathy and support
which they offered her, a few stayed away.

Caring for someone who has AIDS

- Clean up blood or other body fluids *immediately* using household bleach diluted one in ten with water.
- Tissues, plasters or dressings used by someone with AIDS should be burnt or put in a sealed plastic bag and disposed of safely.
- Wear disposable rubber gloves when cleaning up body fluids or handling soiled linen or clothing.
- Laundry should be washed in hot water. Add household bleach diluted one part in ten parts water if linen or clothing is soiled with blood or bodily secretions.
- Do not share needles or other equipment for injecting drugs.
- Do not use the same toothbrush or razor.
- Wash your hands thoroughly with soap and warm water whenever coming into contact with body fluids of a person with AIDS. Cover any cuts or grazes with a waterproof plaster.
- If you have sex make it *safe*! Follow the risk-reduction guidelines described in Chapter Four and, for lesbians, Chapter Three.

There were a couple of people in our neighbourhood who didn't bother to come round, even though they knew Bill was sick. They were afraid. It's the fear of the unknown I think, of contamination, that they might get something. That makes me very, very angry. I suppose it's a matter of educating them, letting them know that they're not going to get it.

The fear of 'catching' AIDS is something that carers of people with AIDS may also experience. A woman whose husband or lover has AIDS, for instance, is particularly likely to feel anxious. Not only will she most likely be worried about what will happen to her partner, but she will also be thinking, 'Will I get it?' In some cases the stresses this can put on a relationship may be too much, and it may end. Alternatively, the experience of dealing with these sorts of anxieties may, in other situations, bring two people closer together.

It is important that lovers, as well as friends and relatives of people with AIDS, have the opportunity to discuss their anxieties about what a diagnosis of AIDS means and the risk of infection to themselves. They need to know what precautions they should take. They also need to be aware of what is likely to happen, both physically and psychologically, to someone who has AIDS as the disease progresses, and of what they can do to help. Bereavement counselling is also often needed.

The possibility of contracting the virus was something that never worried either Maggie or Joyce. They both knew enough about AIDS to understand that, with a few simple precautions, caring for their sons did not put them at risk. (Some of the precautions you should take if you are caring for someone with AIDS are listed on the opposite page.)

In Joyce's case her fears were of losing Bill and how she would cope with this.

> I did think 'Am I going to be able to handle it?' Because I couldn't think of Bill not being there, we'd always been so close to one another. I was afraid I was going to fold, that I wouldn't be able to carry it through. I was fighting that. I was also afraid that my own health would let me down and that my legs would give out on me. I was so completely exhausted.

Many women have a tendency to ignore their own needs while they focus on caring for others. It's important that they have access to people who are supportive of them. Without this they may find the strain of caring for someone who is seriously ill almost too much. Family and friends may be able to provide some of this. It may also be helpful to talk to someone who is going, or has gone, through a similar experience.

Counselling for families, friends and lovers is available at some hospitals and STD clinics (see pages 188–189). A woman who is, or may end up, caring for someone with AIDS may also find it useful to join a self-help group.

Though she says she probably wouldn't go along until her son's condition became much worse, Maggie feels it would help her to talk to women in a similar situation.

Although one thinks one is staunchly independent there are all sorts of things I realise I need. I do need support. Also, you want to know what's going on for other people and, you know, one's weaknesses are not so crushing if you find someone else is just as weak.

Despite the support she received from her family and friends, Joyce also felt this:

I needed to know how to handle this, how to cope with things, what to expect. The doctor could tell me so much, but it wasn't the same; he was a professional. I wanted somebody on my level that I could talk to. Finally, someone put me in touch with the Mothers of AIDS Patients group, so I rang them and went along to a meeting. I came away feeling so wonderfully uplifted to think that I wasn't alone, that it wasn't some curse that had been put on my family, or my son, or on me and my husband. It was something that other people had either gone through or were going through, and that we could battle against together. From that moment on I never felt like I was alone and this was emotionally very stabilising for me.

Mothers of AIDS Patients (MAP) is a self-help and support group for women in the Los Angeles area whose children have AIDS or have died from the disease. In addition to acting as 'penpals' to mothers in other parts of the country, MAP members also work with AIDS patients, becoming, in some cases, 'surrogate mothers' to people

How can I help if someone I know has AIDS?

First of all you can find out about AIDS. Some people with AIDS, or who are antibody positive, have lost friends because they are misinformed or do not understand about how the virus is transmitted. Because they may be afraid of losing friends, a person who has HIV or AIDS needs to know who they can rely on. It is important to reassure them that you are not afraid and that you know you can't get AIDS by simply befriending someone who has it. There are many ways of doing this. For instance Maggie's daughter 'took the children when she visited Richard because she wanted to reassure him that she had no fears of him'. It is also important to show affection and to touch. Like anyone else, someone who is antibody positive or has AIDS needs physical contact and will enjoy the reassurance that goes with it. Remember people with AIDS are *living* with AIDS. Almost every person diagnosed with AIDS is determined to get well again. Use the term 'people with AIDS'. Don't call them a 'victim' of AIDS. This implies they are helpless.

The fear many people have of AIDS is likely to have a big impact on a person's self-esteem and confidence. They may be reluctant to tell others they have AIDS, or the virus which causes it, or to discuss their diagnosis. Show them that if they want to talk about their illness you are willing to listen. Try to understand if they become angry and frustrated, and don't be afraid to talk about how you feel. What is important is that someone who has AIDS has friends with whom they feel they can be honest and at ease.

When someone is not well they may not always feel up to talking. Try to be aware of this and the limits that being ill, as well as often feeling miserable and depressed, can put on a person's social life. Let them know when you intend to visit and don't be offended if they don't want you to stay for very long. People who are ill often tire easily.

People with AIDS progress through their illness at vastly different rates and with varying degrees of ability to continue their daily activities. Offer practical help if you are able, and if you can't visit try to phone or write. If your friend has children, offer to help care for them. Most importantly, *keep in touch*.

with AIDS whose families have rejected them or who have no one coming to visit them.

The need for support groups is more acute for women living in parts of the country where there have so far been relatively few AIDS cases. A woman may also feel isolated for other reasons. For instance, some mothers are not comfortable being in a mixed group for 'significant others'.

Many AIDS organisations, and some hospitals, now have support groups for people caring for someone with AIDS. For information about those and other organisations giving information and advice about AIDS see pages 184–194.

Caring means work

Caring for someone who has AIDS can be hard work. Although people with AIDS may experience periods of relatively good health during which they are able to continue their daily activities, there will also be times when they cannot manage by themselves. Basic everyday tasks such as cooking a meal, shopping, cleaning and doing the laundry have to be done for them. They may be bedridden, especially in the latter stages of the disease, too ill or too weak to wash, feed themselves or even go to the bathroom alone. They may also have dependent children who need looking after.

Usually it is women – as sisters, daughters, wives, mothers, grandmothers, and friends – who are expected to provide this care. The medical profession, social services and the person who is ill may all assume this. They may also take it for granted that however difficult the circumstances a woman will cope. Very rarely are women asked if they feel able to take on board the care of a sick or elderly relative. Nor are they usually asked what help and support they will need to enable them to do the job of caring.

Because of these expectations women, unlike men, can be under considerable pressure to give up a job to care for someone. Women who do give up paid work to become a full-time carer may find it extremely difficult to adjust to being financially dependent on someone else or on state benefits. They may also experience considerable isolation, especially if very few people know about the diagnosis. Equally the strain on women who, by choice or necessity, combine going out to work with providing this kind of physical care can be enormous. Apart from the demands on her time and energy, a woman may feel very anxious or guilty about continuing work.

Jennie goes out to work to support herself and her son, who is in his early thirties and has AIDS. At times, she finds this frustrating:

> I am a single parent, and I do have to go out to work. My son is presently at a time when he does not need a nurse with him at all times. But he does need someone to come in to make sure that he has his lunch, because otherwise he just doesn't want to eat anything. Unfortunately, I don't have any source of any kind to turn to and have someone to come in and do that. That I find frustrating.

The provision of services such as home helps and meals on wheels could reduce the stresses experienced by women caring for people with AIDS, whether working outside the home or not. Day care centres and short-term places in residential homes and hospices would allow care-givers, who may be emotionally drained, the chance to recharge their batteries. Although women's access to such services will vary, many women will not get the practical support they need.

For women who, like Maggie, do want to provide care in the home but who also recognise that they may need some help, this is an important issue.

> I would like to see an availability, a possibility of getting help in the home, most decidedly I would. I think it's terrible if they can't be coped with at home. Basically it

should just be a part of health care. It should be as easy to get help when it's necessary whether it's AIDS or anything else, but it's not likely to be because of the fear of it, in the home anyway, and of course in some hospitals too. It will have to have vast resources allocated to it.

In the present climate the provision of services which would adequately meet the needs of people with AIDS and those who care for them seems unlikely. Despite the fact that this government has repeatedly spoken of the importance of 'care in the community', it has consistently cut back spending on health and social services. Apart from the effects these cutbacks have on women caring for people with AIDS as 'a labour of love', they place an increasing strain on those whose job it is to care.

Women doing AIDS work

Health workers will have to confront their own feelings of sorrow and hopelessness which can result from working with the fatally ill. While most of us develop a certain acceptance of death in the elderly and infirm, few people find it easy to deal with a young person who is dying. The fact that AIDS is a disfiguring and debilitating disease makes it even harder to accept.

The risk of infection is something else which those who provide care for people with AIDS, or the much larger number who are antibody positive, are likely to be concerned about. This is an understandable concern given the nature of the disease. Nevertheless, it would seem that the risk is extremely low. There has not been a single case of a doctor, nurse or hospital technician developing AIDS as a result of working with AIDS patients.

The most likely way in which HIV may be transmitted to medical and nursing staff is through needle-stick injury. Though there are cases of this happening, the risk of infection from such accidents seems to be low. Studies indicate that in almost all cases where hospital staff have accidentally stuck themselves with needles used on people infected with HIV, or who accidentally got blood or other body fluids from AIDS patients splashed on open cuts or sores, the antibody test is negative

Although the evidence is that HIV is not easily transmitted to those who care for people with AIDS, certain precautions do need to be taken.

The main precautions are those which are necessary to avoid coming into contact with bodily fluids. There is no need, for instance, for hospital staff to wear gloves and masks just to enter an AIDS patient's room, as has sometimes happened, or when providing routine care. Masks are necessary only when a patient has a lung infection, such as tuberculosis, or is at risk of catching an infection from you.

Guidelines for health care workers have been drawn up outlining ways of reducing the risk of infection. (In the UK for example, see the report of the Advisory Committee on Dangerous Pathogens, 1986 and the Report of the Royal College of Nursing AIDS Working Party, 1986. In 1988 in Australia, the Commonwealth Department of Community Services and Health AIDS Task Force have published Infection Control Guidelines for AIDS and related conditions.) Among the measures recommended is the careful handling of needles and sharp instruments. The majority of self-inoculation accidents can be avoided by not resheathing needles. Needles should either be thrown away on the syringe or, if this is not possible, removed from syringes without resheathing them and disposed of in a puncture-resistant container. Where there is a risk of coming into contact with blood or other bodily fluids which may contain the virus, disposable rubber gloves and a plastic apron should be worn. The membranes of the eyes and mouth may allow transmission of the virus, and where there is a risk of splashing fluids which may contain HIV, it is advisable to wear goggles and masks.

In addition to knowing about the nature of the disease,

how HIV is transmitted and how the risk of this happening can be reduced, health care workers also need to be aware of the psychological implications of being diagnosed as having AIDS. This is especially true for nurses. Because they are more closely involved with patients, they have a potentially important role to play in providing emotional support as well as physical care.

This can be stressful. Most likely, someone who has AIDS will feel depressed and anxious. They may need to talk about their illness, including their fears about death and dying. They may also feel very angry about the effects of having AIDS, and may take out their anger and frustration on hospital staff. This may also be true of relatives and friends who, in addition, may ask difficult and often upsetting questions. A nurse may have to confront issues that she has never had to deal with before such as, for instance, her own and other people's reactions to gay relationships.

Training programmes for people providing AIDS-related services, both paid and voluntary, should include information and advice on how to deal with these kinds of situations. Also, in addition to developing an understanding of the needs of people with AIDS and those affected by the diagnosis, it may be useful for workers to examine their own attitudes towards death and dying. In view of the fact that, so far in the UK, the majority of those who have developed AIDS are gay men, it is also important to have some knowledge of gay lifestyles. Negative attitudes and judgments regarding gay lifestyles are not uncommon, and will need to be challenged. Health workers should also realise that many AIDS patients experience painful consequences when entering a health care system designed for and administered by a predominantly heterosexual population. Visiting regulations, for instance, may not recognise gay relationships as being as important as other relationships. Wherever possible hospital staff should take steps to prevent this and other forms of discrimination from occurring.

Discrimination can have other implications for care providers. Many gay and bisexual men are careful who they tell about their sexuality. It is vitally important therefore that staff remember who does and does not know. Even when someone is not gay, the stigma surrounding AIDS makes confidentiality a major issue. Those working with people who have AIDS, other HIV-related illness, or who are antibody positive should not disclose information about diagnosis unless the person wants or has agreed to this. The issue of confidentiality is discussed in more detail on page 173.

The stresses on women caring for people with AIDS are made worse by consistent underspending within the health and social services. Without the money to provide more services and with ever-growing numbers of AIDS patients, those whose job it is to provide physical and psychological care come under increasing pressure.

It may be helpful to have a support group for those working with people with AIDS where there is the opportunity to discuss some of the stresses, as well as the practical problems, that can arise. What is really needed, however, is a change in governmental policy to meet the growing costs of AIDS.

Caring for children with AIDS

Although AIDS cases involving children make up only a small percentage of cases reported, an increasing number of babies are being born infected with the virus which causes the disease. As of October 1988, a total of 30 children with AIDS have been reported in the UK. In Australia 9 cases of AIDS in children under the age of 9 years have been reported (by the same date). In the United States the situation is more serious. The CDC reported 1,202 AIDS cases among children younger than 13 (by this date). In 941 cases, mothers were HIV positive, 156 were infected by blood transfusions, 71 were haemophiliacs who had received infected blood products and 34 cases were of undetermined cause. The incidence of AIDS in black and Hispanic children is much higher than for white children – 53 per cent of these children were black and 23 per cent Hispanic.

Because screening methods for blood and blood products now exist, most future cases of AIDS in children are likely to occur in infants whose mothers are infected. At present, more than three-quarters of the children with AIDS in the United States acquired the virus from their mothers during pregnancy or at birth. It is not yet known what proportion of children who contract the virus from their mothers are likely to go on to develop AIDS, though some doctors have suggested that it may be as many as half.

The other main way in which children have got AIDS is through receiving a transfusion with infected blood or blood products. This includes children with haemophilia – almost all of whom are male – who received treatment with the blood clotting agents factor 8 and factor 9. Of the 700 or so children who have haemophilia in the UK most have now been tested for antibodies to HIV. About a third are antibody positive. In Australia it is estimated that between a quarter to a third of children who received factor 8 before screening was introduced in May 1985 are HIV positive, although in Western Australia the figure is lower due mainly to the use of blood donated there. (Most people diagnosed with AIDS or who are HIV positive in Australia reside in Eastern states, in particular New South Wales.)

The risk of this happening in future has been eliminated through the screening of blood donors and heat treatment of blood products. The number of children with haemophilia who are infected with HIV will therefore gradually diminish as these children grow up.

There are other reasons why a child may become infected with HIV and develop AIDS. Children who have been sexually abused may have been infected by the abuser. Also, older children may be sexually active, or experimenting with injectable drugs, in ways that put them at risk.

There is little research as yet on children with AIDS and how to treat them. Often, infected children will develop at a normal rate during their first months, but then fail to grow and decline in health. The symptoms seen most often in paediatric AIDS include pneumonia, lymphadenopathy and persistent diarrhoea. Persistent and recurrent thrush in the mouth and failure to thrive are also very common, although Kaposi's sarcoma is rare.

Many women have no idea prior to their children's diagnosis that they are infected. They have to deal with not only the shock of finding out that their infant has a fatal illness, caused by a virus which they transmitted, but also that they themselves could develop AIDS and die. Even if they are prepared for the news, being told that their child has AIDS or the virus which can lead to it will still be enormously distressing for most women. Mothers of children with AIDS must deal with the fact that their child may very likely die soon.

If their child does become ill and develops AIDS they may feel very guilty that it is their fault. (This may apply to mothers of children with haemophilia as well as, more obviously, to women who have transmitted the virus to their infants. Knowing that she is a carrier of haemophilia, a woman may blame herself for passing on the disease which has put her child at risk.)

This may be exacerbated by the reactions of others who cannot understand why they got pregnant or continued with the pregnancy if they knew about their own antibody status. This lack of understanding is rooted in an inability to see the situation from the perspective of the woman. How far is getting pregnant or continuing with the pregnancy a choice? Apart from access to contraception and abortion, becoming a mother is tremendously important to many women.

Some women will be anxious about other people finding out that their child is antibody positive or has AIDS. One of the reasons for not wanting anyone to know is in case their child becomes stigmatised. Some parents, fearing that their own child might be at risk of infection, have demanded that children with HIV be removed from schools or daycare. Similarly, other children might refuse to mix or play with a child who is known to be infected with the virus.

Children with AIDS often suffer the same stigmatisation as adults with the disease. However, in the United States the situation is compounded by the fact that 76 per cent of children with AIDS are black or Hispanic, and that often their parents are IV drug users who themselves may be ill or dying from AIDS.

Women who have AIDS or are antibody positive and have children may have other worries. A common fear is that they will lose custody of their children or be unable to care for them. In general, it is women who are expected to care for children. But since most cases of AIDS in young children are the result of maternal transmission, the mother may herself be ill and unable to care full-time for her children. The burden of care may then fall on the grand-mother. In the United States, however, many children with AIDS spend their entire lives in hospitals, even when they are healthy enough to be discharged, because their mothers are ill or have died of AIDS and there is no one else to care for them. Access to childcare, and housing programmes for people with AIDS which accept children, would make it possible for these women to keep their children much longer.

Fostering also has a role to play. Foster parents could be used as respite carers, giving the mother a break from the demands of caring for a child with AIDS as well as, in some cases, a partner who has the disease.

The foster family will have to come to terms with the demands of short-term care and becoming attached to a young child whose long-term prognosis is poor and whose life-span is likely to be short. Fostering older children or adolescents who are infected or at risk presents other issues. They may want information about their condition and the effects that HIV will have. They will also need advice about sex and drug use and may need help in dealing with AIDS discrimination and prejudice they encounter. Foster parents therefore need to be well-informed about AIDS in order that they can deal with the issue at the young person's pace, whenever they want to talk. They also need to be prepared for questions such as 'Am I going to die?' Like any other family caring for a child with AIDS or HIV infection, they will need counselling about helping the child to deal with his or her feelings, as well as bereavement counselling and help with coping with their own emotional reactions. They may also need access to respite care.

Confidentiality is a major issue with regard to AIDS and fostering. Great consideration is needed in deciding who needs to know that the foster child is infected and why. Because of the possibility of AIDS-related discrimination only those who really need to know should be told about the child's condition – such as the child's doctor who *ought*, in any case, to respect confidentiality.

Clearly, foster parents should be informed if they are to look after a child with AIDS or who is antibody positive. But some parents may not know their child is infected, or may not say so in an effort to prevent their child from being rejected by potential foster or adoptive parents. One way of trying to overcome this would be to routinely test *all* children for HIV antibodies before adoption or fostering. However, the British Agencies for Adoption and Fostering has denounced this in terms both of the ethical issues it raises and, also, because it is extemely difficult to test infants under a year old accurately.

There are a number of other policy issues to consider with regard to fostering and adoption of children with AIDS or who are HIV antibody positive. For example, if a child is known to be infected should a potential foster family include other children? Ordinary social contact does not put non-infected children at risk, but the increased risk of colds and illness to a young infected child may lead local authorities to avoid placing such children in a household with other very young children. Equally it can be argued that contact with other children is essential for social and emotional development.

It is important that parents, as well as teachers, understand that children are not at risk of getting AIDS through normal social contact with other children, such as occurs in school or day care. There have been no cases of young children getting AIDS from other children. Children who have brothers and sisters with AIDS have played, eaten, slept, kissed and fought with them without getting the virus. Even if a child gets bitten, this is unlikely to transmit the virus. In one case a man with ARC, who had been brain damaged due to an automobile accident, bit and scratched thirty health care workers. All thirty when tested were antibody negative. Similarly, even if a child with AIDS or HIV is cut or injured, routine safety procedures for handling blood or other bodily fluids – which should apply to all children in school or day care – will prevent transmission.

In addition to parents educating their children about AIDS, schools should make sure that both staff and pupils know how HIV is transmitted. Some children may be at risk. Others may be unnecessarily worried about getting AIDS. Children need to know that people with AIDS, including other children, are not contagious. They also need to know that just because someone is gay, for instance, does *not* mean that they will get AIDS.

Teachers and day care staff need to be aware of the importance of maintaining confidentiality. They *should tell no one* that a child is sero-positive, or has AIDS, unless they have permission from the child's parents to do so. Most haemophilia centres do not tell schools which of the children they treat are antibody positive. They take the view that teachers should know, in any case, how to deal with a bleeding injury if a child in their care is known to have haemophilia and, possibly, HIV.

Deciding what to tell a child with AIDS about their condition is a difficult decision to make. It will depend on many factors, such as the age of the child and how ill they are. The decision not to tell others may also be difficult to

---

Caring for children who are antibody positive or have AIDS

- Any spills of blood should be cleaned up using household bleach diluted one in ten with water.
- Urine, faeces and vomit may contain blood. Wear disposable rubber gloves when cleaning these up, and cover any cuts on your hands with waterproof plasters.
- Carers should use disposable rubber gloves when changing and handling soiled nappies.
- Dirty nappies should be burnt, flushed down the toilet or put in a sealed plastic bag and disposed of safely. Non-disposable nappies and clothes or linen that are stained with blood, urine, vomit or faeces should be washed in the hottest cycle of a washing machine or boiled.
- Because the virus is transmitted in blood it is important to discourage practices such as tattooing and ear-piercing, which some children may engage in. Cover any cuts or grazes on either yourself or your child with waterproof plasters.
- It may be dangerous for children with HIV infection to have vaccinations which use live virus, such as oral polio vaccine. Also, the immunisation of healthy children and adults in the household of a child with AIDS can pose a risk. Carers should seek medical advice before having either their child or themselves vaccinated.
- Children with AIDS or HIV infection should not share their toothbrushes with others, because gums often bleed during brushing.
- Children with AIDS or who are antibody positive have the same need for affection as other children. There is no risk in hugging or cuddling them.

---

explain to a child. As one woman said, 'it's hard to explain to them that although having HIV or AIDS is nothing to be ashamed of, this is something to be kept a secret.'

Children who are antibody positive or have AIDS need to

have as normal a life as possible. If a child is unable to control bodily wastes or has oozing lesions (which cannot be covered) she may not be able to attend school or day care. But in many cases, providing they are in good health, there is no reason for children with AIDS to be isolated in the home. They have the same needs for play and stimulation as other children. They need friendship and affection, not isolation from others. Some HIV infected children may develop impaired mental functions, in which case special educational provision may be required. Otherwise at school they should be treated in the same way as other pupils.

There are a few precautions which someone caring for a child with HIV infection or AIDS needs to take. Some of these are listed on the previous page. Since children with AIDS are highly susceptible to infections, much of the emphasis on hygiene is to protect the child. Further information on reducing the risk of infection, especially within schools, is contained in the DES booklet *Children at School: Problems Related to AIDS*.

Women whose children have AIDS are likely to require services that often do not exist, such as foster and day care programmes and support groups for mothers of young children with AIDS. Health and social service providers are beginning to deal with these issues. The following chapter examines this and other aspects of AIDS policy-making in more detail, and asks the question, 'What can be done?'

7   Policies and prevention

Policy makers have, until recently, done little to halt the spread of AIDS. Undoubtedly, if AIDS had initially affected a different social group than gay men then the situation would have been different. However, as long as the disease is confined largely to certain groups – gay men and IV drug users, and in the US, black and Hispanic women – governments do very little. It is only the recognition that AIDS poses a threat to the (white) heterosexual as well as the gay community that has prompted governments to take AIDS more seriously and, alongside this, provide more funding.

Funding nevertheless remains an urgent priority, especially for the treatment and care of those who have already been infected with HIV. In addition to providing more money for AIDS programmes, the government must also examine the wider social implications of AIDS – in particular, the need for legislation to prevent discrimination against people with AIDS, or who are antibody positive, in employment, health care delivery, housing, education, and child custody.

Education

The three major areas which need funding are prevention campaigns, health and social service programmes for people with AIDS, and research aimed at developing a cure and vaccine. In the United States the major focus of government funding so far has been research, in particular on finding a vaccine to protect people who do not have AIDS from getting it. The government has neglected to provide adequate funding either for the medical treatment and care of those who are ill or dying from AIDS or other HIV-related illness, or for education.

The British experience is a few years behind that of the United States. We therefore have the opportunity to learn from their mistakes, and to take steps to try to prevent the AIDS epidemic from reaching the same proportions here.

Clearly, it was a mistake that education was the least well planned component of AIDS prevention measures in the United States. A vaccine has not yet been developed and probably won't be until the 1990s at the earliest. Even if a vaccine is produced, it may not offer the ultimate solution. One of the characteristics of HIV is that it is constantly changing and producing new strains. A vaccine which is effective against one strain may not be against another. (Some of the problems in developing a vaccine are discussed on page 25.)

In the absence of a vaccine or a cure, public education is the most effective way of preventing AIDS. Apart from the human suffering which AIDS causes, attempts to halt the disease also make good economic sense when one considers the cost of providing AIDS-related services. AIDS is an expensive illness to treat. Thousands of pounds spent on education now could save millions of pounds on medical treatment and care in the future.

However, what we must remember is that AIDS unites things which society is reluctant to talk about: homosexuality, sexual disease, drug use and death. In addition to this, the much-needed explicit advice about safe sex may be resisted because it involves discussing activities that some people consider immoral or offensive.

In the United States concern about how the public would react to widespread discussion of, in particular, homosexuality and drug use has fundamentally influenced attitudes towards education campaigns. In Los Angeles, for

example, the State Department of Health Services issued a
directive to halt distribution of an AIDS prevention brochure aimed at gay men. The pamphlet, *Mother's Handy Sex
Guide*, advised gay men about safer sex practices and was
part of the 'LA Cares' mass media campaign launched in
1985. Another brochure aimed at encouraging gay men to
adopt safer sexual practices was attacked by a Los Angeles
county supervisor as 'hard core pornographic trash, totally
unsuitable for the public'. Such responses culminated, in
1987, in the United States senate voting overwhelmingly to
stop federal funds for AIDS programmes which 'promote
or encourage, directly or indirectly, "homosexual activities",' after a federal-funded book, produced by New York
Gay Men's Health Crisis, showed safer sex between two
men.

There has been similar resistance to AIDS education
aimed at telling IV drug users how to inject drugs safely. In
this case the concern is that this condones drug use.

If we in Britain are to learn anything from such reactions,
it is that they should be avoided at all costs. The only way
for individuals to protect themselves from getting AIDS is
to know how HIV may be transmitted and to take steps to
reduce the risk of this happening. For some this will mean
a significant change in social and sexual attitudes. AIDS
education, if it is to be effective, must tackle this. It must,
for example, challenge the widely held belief, especially
amongst men, that every road to ultimate sexual satisfaction must end in intercourse – this is a way of transmitting
the virus.

A good example of public education on AIDS is found in
San Francisco. The city's programme includes advertisements on public transport and TV and in newspaper
and magazines, and news and feature stories, as well as
explicit leaflets for those at risk. While the efforts of voluntary organisations such as the San Francisco AIDS Foundation and the Shanti Project have been enormously important, such developments also reflect the willingness of the
city government to become involved in attempts to prevent

the spread of AIDS. San Francisco has provided more direct support to AIDS programmes than any other city in the United States.

Australia has a strong tradition of public health initiatives, usually done through television. During February 1987, the government launched a series of TV advertisements about AIDS which coincided with newspapers and magazines providing information sections on AIDS.

In Britain, the government was initially slow to respond to the need for educational programmes aimed at preventing people from developing AIDS. Until 1986, the provision of information was left largely to voluntary organisations such as the Terrence Higgins Trust and the Haemophilia Society. Towards the end of 1986, however, following criticism of a newspaper campaign in the spring of that year, the government launched a £20 million information campaign to combat AIDS. The campaign, entitled 'AIDS: Don't Die of Ignorance', included advertisements on billboards and radio, as well as in newspapers and magazines. In the New Year commercials about AIDS reached our television and cinema screens, and leaflets advising people how to avoid infection with HIV were distributed to each of Britain's 23 million homes. Media attention culminated in a week of saturation coverage on all four television channels during 'AIDS week' in February 1987.

As a start, this was a welcome sign that at last the government was beginning to take AIDS prevention seriously. But the government will in future have to do much more to ensure that people understand about AIDS and how HIV is transmitted. (For instance, such a campaign does not reach the illiterate, the homeless, or those who can't speak or read its language.) What is needed is a variety of campaigns directed at different groups, in easily understood language, that is ethnically and culturally relevant to those it is aimed at.

Different communities will have different cultural beliefs about illness, death, and sexuality. They will also have different voices of authority on these matters. For instance, as a credible source within certain sections of the black community, church leaders are in a position to play an important role in AIDS education. Similarly, AIDS prevention campaigns aimed at Catholic communities will need to be sensitive to the powerful influence of the Church.

We also need AIDS education campaigns specifically aimed at women – in particular, women who inject drugs, black women, lesbians, prostitutes, and women considering pregnancy.

The government's AIDS campaign has also been criticised for using scare tactics. For instance, linking AIDS with images of gravestones or, as in Australia, depicting AIDS as the 'grim reaper', does little to dispel people's anxieties and irrational fears about the disease.

Educational programmes are essential to any prevention effort, but they will not be enough by themselves. What is also needed are ways to motivate people to act on the information they have. It is not enough, for instance, to tell people they should 'always use a condom.' Also needed are ways to help people to make changes in their sexual practices. Condoms should be free and more easily available through chemists, doctor's surgeries, family planning and STD clinics, supermarkets and public toilets. It has also been suggested that they should be freely available in schools and in prisons.

The government's campaign, and recent mass media coverage about AIDS, seems to have been successful in communicating the basic facts about AIDS. However, it is also apparent from studies that have been carried out that many people are still uncertain about how AIDS affects them. In particular people want to know how exactly they could reduce the risk to themselves. This especially applies to women. As I have already pointed out, women may have particular problems in getting their partners to agree to safer sex. It is vital that educators recognise that, for women, AIDS prevention is often as much about developing a sense of empowerment as it is about having access to information. No amount of AIDS education or assertiveness training will change the reality for women of their social and economic situation. In this sense what is required is not so much educational intervention as major social changes in the relationship of women to men.

Apart from the further funding of materials which attempt to resolve people's concerns about AIDS, what we also need is a change in educational policy towards the teaching of human sexuality. In most schools and colleges sex education is based around discussions of human reproduction, with little if any discussion of lesbian and gay lifestyles or other ways of being sexual besides vaginal intercourse. Although it specifically excludes initiatives for the prevention of AIDS, the section of the Local Government Act which, since May 1988, has made it illegal for a local authority to intentionally 'promote' homosexuality or promote in State schools the teaching of homosexuality as a 'pretended family relationship', is unlikely to foster a climate in which teachers feel able to talk openly about the realities of human sexual experience, in all its complexity and diversity.

Young people must be given information about AIDS and how HIV is transmitted so that they become aware of the risks associated with certain kinds of sex and, also, of experimenting with injecting drugs. Children also need to know that having AIDS, or being antibody positive, 'doesn't mean that you are a bad person', or that you are contagious and to be avoided.

Others have suggested abstinence and would oppose such educational developments on the grounds that it would encourage children to be sexual or take drugs. Abstinence may seem like a simple and effective solution – but it's unrealistic. It's foolish to believe that if children don't know about something they won't do it. Many teenagers are sexually active and experiment with drugs. Information about sex and drugs will help them to make safer and more responsible decisions about what they do. Sex education in schools is therefore vital, and must include explicit discussion of sexuality in the broadest sense.

Under the Education Act, which came into effect in September 1987, it is school governors who now have the powers to determine what sex education there should be in schools. (The Act also gives parents the right to decide whether their child receives sex education in school.) Teachers, parents and school governors have an opportunity to consider how education about sexuality and AIDS might lead not only to the prevention of AIDS but also to greater understanding and honesty about sex. It would be unfortunate if, given their new responsibilities, they failed to respond to what are important educational needs.

AIDS education is essential not only as a form of disease prevention, but also as a means of combating the fear and ignorance surrounding the disease. This, in combination with racist, sexist and anti-gay attitudes, helps explain why some people with AIDS have experienced a hostile or unsympathetic response from others. The mass media, which has a potentially important role to play in AIDS education, must take some responsibility for this. Indeed, the approach of certain sections of the media has been both sensationalising and judgmental. This kind of media coverage has done absolutely nothing to allay people's irrational fears, in particular that AIDS is a casually spread disease. It is not.

It is vital that this is widely understood, especially by those who have to care for people with AIDS. Yet even amongst social service and health care workers it would appear that fears about contracting HIV through routine contact with AIDS patients do exist. Such fears can result in decreased quality of care to people with AIDS. Home helps have refused to enter the homes of people with AIDS; other staff have been reluctant to deliver meals on wheels. There have, in the past, also been cases of hospital staff refusing to feed or wash a patient if they have AIDS. Similarly, some doctors have told their patients not to come back to their surgery if they have AIDS.

Such examples only serve to underline the importance of providing educational programmes for social service and health care workers of all grades. More generally, it is essential that we all learn to recognise the *real* risks of getting AIDS and how to protect ourselves against them.

Health and Social Services

Health education is not the only AIDS-related policy issue that we need to consider. The provision of funds for health and social services programmes for those with AIDS and HIV-related conditions is also a major area of concern, particularly as the number of cases of AIDS continues to grow.

Despite this, the health and social service needs of people with AIDS have not been considered funding priorities. On the contrary, the health and social services have found themselves having to cope with AIDS at a time when the Thatcher government is committed to making major cuts in spending. Apart from the strain this has placed on the medical and welfare services that already exist, this has had direct effects on the care and treatment of people with AIDS.

The situation will worsen as more people develop AIDS, unless the government provides funding for the expansion of services that are urgently needed. This has particular implications for women. The health system is already biased against the needs of women, especially those who are poor, black, or who may possibly be at risk of AIDS through injecting drugs. This is especially true of the United States where almost three-quarters of the women who have AIDS are black or latina. The greater poverty experienced by these women means that they are, in general, far less able to obtain good medical care or to seek medical attention early on. Many Hispanics are frightened to go to the doctor because of the fear of divulging their legal residency status in the United States. As a result, they die sooner after diagnosis than white AIDS patients. The average life span of a white person with AIDS in the United

States is two years. A black or latina person with AIDS is expected to live, on average, between four and five months.

Improved care and access to support, both in and out of hospital, is alongside housing perhaps the most pressing need for AIDS patients. In the case of hospital and medical care of people with AIDS this means more hospital beds, more equipment and more staff to meet the increased workload generated by AIDS patients.

An alternative to hospital care is the kind of care offered by the hospice movement to the terminally ill. Hospice care could play an increasingly important role in the care and treatment of people with AIDS. Again, this will depend on whether funding is available. At present, hospice care for people with AIDS is very limited.

Further government spending on the training of health workers in caring for people with AIDS is also needed. Research on the development of therapies to treat those who have already been infected with HIV also remains in urgent need of government support.

Apart from hospital care, which is enormously costly, more support services are needed to enable people with AIDS to be cared for at home if that is what they want. A person with AIDS may be too ill to cook a meal for themselves or do the housework or shopping. They may not even be able to get out of bed on their own. Home-help programmes and improved hospital out-patients services are therefore necessary, if people with AIDS are to be cared for within the community. More health and social workers trained in counselling people with AIDS will also be needed to provide emotional support and help when dealing with the many difficult issues that a diagnosis of AIDS, or an HIV antibody positive result, raises. This will include dealing with the reactions of friends, family and lovers.

At present, the National Health Service is severely strained in caring for the sick. As the numbers of people with AIDS grow, this is likely to place a greater burden for AIDS care on the 'community'. As I have already pointed out, what this often means is women providing the care.

All too often social policy makers, in arguing for community care, fail to acknowledge this. This must not happen with AIDS. Arguments for community care policies for people with AIDS must recognise the costs to carers, especially where few support services for carers are available. There may be good grounds for caring for people with AIDS within the community, but this must not be at the expense, or exploitation, of women.

Apart from caring for the sick and the elderly, the role of caring for children is a traditional one for women. While this may be a very rewarding experience, for some women the conditions in which they have to care for children can mean stress, exhaustion, loneliness or boredom. Such feelings very often arise from the tremendous responsibility attached to being a mother. This reflects men's lack of involvement in child care. It also highlights the lack of social service provision for women with young children, in particular the provision of adequate day care facilities.

Women who have children with AIDS are likely to find caring for their children particularly stressful. This will be especially true of those women who themselves have AIDS or other HIV-related illness. A woman who is too ill to care of her children may be forced to have them taken into care or fostered. Alternatively, women who are still healthy but have passed the virus on to their child may have to deal with their child developing AIDS and dying.

Children with AIDS create enormous social policy problems concerning day care and schools, as well as fostering and adoption for children whose mothers die or become ill. These are issues which social workers and teachers are increasingly going to have to deal with. In New York, where there are more cases of AIDS in children than anywhere else in the United States, foster and day care programmes for children with AIDS have been developed. Nevertheless, because of the fear of AIDS and an understandable reluctance to care for a child with a terminal illness, many of these children will continue to be difficult to place.

Apart from needing more fostering and day care programmes, as well as better housing and welfare, women with young children are also very often in need of emotional support and help. In the case of women whose children have AIDS, this means providing counselling and other forms of social support.

Counselling and advisory services for those at risk are also needed. Some women may be anxious to know if they have been infected with HIV and will need counselling about whether or not they should take the antibody test. Further counselling will be needed if they decide to take the test and it turns out to be positive. Because of the possible risks to the woman and her child if she were to become pregnant, this should include comprehensive advice about contraception and abortion, as well as ways of reducing the risk of infection to others through safer sex and safer drug use.

At present, voluntary organisations like the Terrence Higgins Trust, the Haemophilia Society and drug advice agencies are helping to meet some of the deficiencies in the health and social service systems as they currently exist. They provide information about AIDS prevention, as well as offering support and counselling to those with AIDS, or who are antibody positive, and their partners, friends and families. The Terrence Higgins Trust, for example, runs support groups for people with AIDS and who are antibody positive. They can also provide 'buddies' for people with AIDS. These are volunteers who provide practical help and emotional support to someone with AIDS, or who is antibody positive, on a regular basis. Body Positive is another self-help organisation, based in London, which runs support groups for people who have taken the HIV antibody test and are positive.

Most of the support groups currently available are for gay or bisexual men. This reflects the fact that so far it is mainly they who have been affected by AIDS. Where support groups for women do exist, these tend to be for women who are caring for someone with AIDS.

As more women develop AIDS it will become necessary to provide counselling and support services for them. While the existence of voluntary support is important and must continue, this needs to be in conjunction with increased spending in the public sector. Even if those who are most affected by AIDS could afford medical insurance, most insurance companies will not provide health or life cover for people with AIDS or who are viewed as 'at risk'. The question then is who is going to pay for the care of people with AIDS?

So far the government has failed to provide adequate funding for the services that are needed for people with AIDS and those who care for them. Already the provision of health and social services is severely challenged by AIDS. As more people become ill they will no longer be able to cope with the demands put on them. It is vital that government planners and policy makers recognise this. What we need, and now, is a comprehensive long-term plan to develop health and social services to care for and support people with AIDS and other HIV-related illness and those looking after them.

Housing

In common with a significant proportion of the population of the United Kingdom, many people with AIDS are dependent on state benefits. In some cases this is because they are too ill to work. In others it is because they have lost their job as a result of their employer finding out they have AIDS. Whatever the reason, such financial hardship is likely to lead to problems with paying a mortgage or rent.

Housing can pose serious difficulties for other reasons. Some people were homeless prior to developing AIDS. Some people with AIDS have been evicted when their landlords have discovered their illness, or have lost their home when their lover, friends or family have refused to continue to support them.

A woman with AIDS, or who is antibody positive, who becomes homeless can apply for local authority housing and be accepted as a priority for housing under the terms of the Housing (Homeless Persons) Act. However, this may not be easy, and in some cases it may take a lot of effort to get the council to do anything. Even then, the kind of accommodation offered may be unsuitable. Very often the homeless are housed in poor quality accommodation, which may be damp or difficult to heat.

It is vital that local authorities become more aware of the housing problems faced by people with AIDS and other HIV-related illness, and provide low-cost or no-cost housing for those who can't afford or find adequate housing. Apart from access to accommodation that is suitable to their needs, it is important that people with AIDS are housed quickly. For this to be possible housing agencies, together with voluntary organisations, need to develop housing programmes with AIDS in mind.

In San Francisco, voluntary organisations like the Shanti Project, with city government money and support, are able to provide low-cost housing for people made homeless through AIDS. Only people with AIDS live in the houses, whose location is kept secret to protect the privacy of those living there. Each person has her or his own bedroom and shares the kitchen, bathroom and living room facilities with the other residents. Shanti also provides home care services for those who are ill to help them stay in their own home rather than go into hospital, if that is what they want.

Women with AIDS are particularly likely to have housing difficulties. While most people with AIDS experience financial hardship, women are more susceptible to this than are men. Women in general earn lower wages and may not be able to afford rent or a mortgage. Also, AIDS affects women who are often already impoverished. In the United States, a disproportionately high number of women with AIDS are black and latina. Add to this the fact that over half of those cases of AIDS in women are among IV drug users and it is easy to see why many women with AIDS become homeless.

Women are also more often the sole supporters of children. Many housing programmes for people with AIDS do not take children or, for that matter, people who are drug dependent. Women may be forced to choose between having a home and keeping their family together. In housing, as in other areas, it is essential that AIDS organisations begin to address the special needs of women affected by AIDS.

The housing problems of those with AIDS or who are antibody positive are not simply about having somewhere stable to live. They are also about being able to choose the kind of accommodation they want. At present, the range of choices available to people with AIDS is very limited. Housing programmes specifically designed to meet the needs of people with AIDS remain in urgent need of government support. Further long-term financing is needed to meet the costs of providing more hospital beds and hospice facilities, as well as out-patient services and community care for those who prefer to remain in their own homes. There is also likely to be a growing demand for mental health hostel places and sheltered housing, associated with the tendency of HIV to cause early dementia, in some cases, due to brain damage.

AIDS discrimination – the antibody test

For what purposes should governments permit the use of blood tests to determine the presence of antibodies to HIV? Should the test be used to screen applicants for medical insurance or for immigration or employment? Should it be used to screen travellers from other countries? (Accusations of racial discrimination were, quite rightly, levelled at the British government in 1986 for suggesting compulsory screening of African visitors to Britain.) If the use of testing is to be promoted for the control of infection, how should this be done? Should people 'at risk' be required to submit to HIV testing?

In the UK the HIV antibody test is used to screen blood that is donated. It is also used to screen semen and donors of kidneys, hearts, livers, etc. In Australia it is also compulsory to take the test if you work in the armed services. (Also, in Queensland, all prisoners are tested, and other states are considering doing the same.) In the United States the test is also used to screen people for certain jobs. For instance, since 1985 all military personnel have been required to take the HIV antibody test. Those already enlisted who are sero-positive have, so far, not been discharged but new recruits who test positive are rejected. More recently, the Reagan administration approved the use of the test in screening immigrants to the United States. In the past year, proposals have also been discussed in several countries regarding the screening of international travellers for HIV antibodies.

Opinions differ as to whether it is appropriate to use the test to screen people. A major concern is that this may lead to new forms of social control of women. Will HIV testing soon become part of routine antenatal care for instance? In some countries, this is already happening. In Norway, for example, more than 71,000 pregnant women have been tested (by August 1988). If a woman refuses to take the test she is treated as if she were positive. The development of a test for antibodies to HIV also makes the introduction of compulsory screening of prostitutes a possibility. Similar fears that the antibody test might be used to single out gay men should also not be regarded as groundless.

A common argument for routine screening is that it would help control the 'spread' of AIDS. Those who were antibody positive could be advised on how to reduce the risk of transmitting the virus to others. The assumption is that a person will be more likely to alter their behaviour if they know whether they are positive or negative than if they do not know. There is no conclusive evidence that testing brings about more behavioural change than education alone. Also, while some people may find it easier to change their lifestyle if they know the test result, the advice is the same whether they are positive or negative: practise safer sex and drug use to avoid contracting the virus and, in the case of those who are sero-positive, passing it on to others. Consequently, many would argue that until an effective treatment or cure for AIDS becomes available there is little to be gained from taking the test.

In the United States the CDC has considered introducing mandatory testing of some individuals including prisoners, prostitutes, those participating in drug programmes, visiting family planning and STD clinics, applying for marriage licences, and pregnant women.

Mandatory testing means you have to take the test. Routine testing means that you are given the test after you have been told that testing will be done. Theoretically, you have the right to refuse. Voluntary testing is where you decide you want to take the test.

The CDC's proposals were overwhelmingly rejected by public health officials from all over the United States at a meeting held in Atlanta, Georgia in February 1987. One argument against mandatory testing is that it would be both expensive and difficult to implement. It could also be medically counterproductive. Those at risk might be driven underground. It could also give a false sense of security to those who tested negative. Without nationwide anti-discrimination and confidentiality legislation for HIV positive individuals and people with AIDS and other HIV-related illness, many are also concerned that mandatory testing would seriously threaten civil rights.

Despite the rejection of the CDC proposals, some states have since introduced 'AIDS laws'. For instance, in parts of the United States couples are now required to take an HIV antibody test before they can apply for a marriage licence. The legislation in each state differs, but so far none restricts the right to marry if you do test positive.

In this country the introduction of 'routine testing' of pregnant women is being talked about. This would mean that the HIV antibody test would be included as one of the standard blood tests given to pregnant women. While taking the test would be voluntary, it would not be with informed consent. Even if a woman was told that the HIV antibody test was one of the tests she would be given and had to give her consent to it being carried out, she may find it difficult to say no. Some women, for example, may be afraid that if they didn't agree to have the tests they wouldn't get the treatment they needed.

There are a number of reasons why women who are at risk, or whose partners are at risk, and are thinking about becoming pregnant or are in the early stages of pregnancy may benefit from taking the test (see pages 58–64). It is therefore important that women are informed about the relationship between pregnancy and AIDS. However, it must remain *their* decision whether or not they take the test.

A more extreme 'AIDS control' measure is the suggestion that people with AIDS, and those having tested positive on the HIV antibody test, could be quarantined. In 1986, in California, followers of Lyndon LaRouche endorsed Proposition 64. This was a cleverly drafted initiative which, interpreted one way, could have forced state health officials to quarantine people with AIDS. The measure was overwhelmingly defeated; however, similar measures are still being discussed both in the US and in other parts of the world.

Given the irrational fears and prejudices which surround AIDS it is perhaps not surprising that the idea of isolating those who have AIDS, or who are antibody positive, should have occurred. However, apart from the ethical objections to quarantine, as a public health measure this is neither realistic nor appropriate. HIV is comparatively difficult to contract and it is hard to see how one could use quarantine when 5,000 people in the UK are already believed to be infected. It is through public education and counselling on safer sex and drug use that the growth in the number of people with AIDS will hopefully be halted.

Another reason for limiting the use of tests is that it can be detrimental for a person to know that they are HIV positive. Many people are shocked by the news and become anxious or depressed. This is why it is essential that counselling is available both before and after the test.

While counselling can often help to overcome psychological difficulties, people who are antibody positive can have other problems. For instance, some people have lost their jobs once it was discovered that they were seropositive. There are then often financial and accommodation problems.

Sometimes people who are antibody positive have been denied medical treatment. Insurance companies are reluctant to give health or life insurance to anyone who is seropositive or thought to be 'at risk'. This can make it difficult to get a mortgage.

The AIDS hysteria generated by the media is partly to blame for this. However, discrimination against people with AIDS and those who are antibody positive is also connected with the fact that in the public imagination AIDS is linked with homosexuality. To a large extent, it is homophobia and anti-lesbianism, not AIDS, that's the root of the problem.

Some American states have passed laws forbidding AIDS-related discrimination. Wisconsin and California specifically forbid discrimination on the basis of the HIV antibody result. It is also illegal in California, as well as certain other states, either to administer the HIV antibody test or to disclose the test results without a person's written permission. In other parts of the country, New York for example, laws prohibiting discriminatory practices against people who have disabilities have been extended to people with AIDS. (It is also illegal in New York to discriminate against a person because you think they may have AIDS.) By contrast, in some states, including Colorado, it is the law that doctors and clinics must report the names of those who test positive to the state department of health. While these lists are said to be confidential there's no knowing how this information might be used in the future.

In the UK, there are at present no laws specifically designed to protect the rights of people with AIDS or those who are antibody positive. (In Australia all states are currently working on the introduction of legislation which would do this.) Under such conditions, confidentiality is a major issue. Many people are tested at STD clinics which are governed by special regulations to guarantee anonymity. These regulations require that, when a disease has been sexually transmitted, a health worker may not disclose information to anyone not involved in the treatment of the patient without their permission. Clinical records are also kept separate from the main hospital records which tend to be less confidential.

Confidentiality is an agreement that information about you will not be disclosed without your consent. Your GP can arrange tests. However, they may not be able to guarantee confidentiality. If a doctor writes your results in your medical records, employers or insurance companies may be able to gain access to this information.

For these reasons, many AIDS organisations recommend that people who decide to take the test should have it done *anonymously*. The advantage of not giving your (real) name is that only you, and the people you decide to tell, will know the result. Where anonymous testing is not possible, the strongest possible guarantee of confidentiality should be obtained from a doctor or clinic.

It is not enough for doctors to say they won't tell anyone if a patient has AIDS or is antibody positive. They should be prohibited by law from releasing names without good reason. Failure to implement measures to ensure confidentiality will mean continued difficulties for people who have AIDS or are antibody positive. Some may even put their lives at risk because they are afraid to go to their doctor in case their virus status becomes known.

At present, given the discrimination which exists towards people with AIDS and who are antibody positive, the use of the HIV antibody test should be carefully controlled. It must be used to screen blood and semen that is donated, as well as body tissue; it must be used for research. But it should not be used to screen people, particularly without their 'informed consent'. (We need to recognise of course that there are all sorts of ways in which someone may feel forced to 'consent'.) Bearing this in mind, the test should be widely and freely available for those who wish to use it. However, it is essential that they be counselled about the social, economic, employment and emotional consequences of a positive test result *before* taking the test.

8 The Challenge of AIDS

AIDS has been used to legitimise many of the fears and prejudices already embedded in our society. Right-wing moralists, for example, regard AIDS as proof that their values are correct. In their view sex outside marriage, and sex with someone of the same sex, is morally wrong. AIDS is a recognition of this, a punishment from God for society's 'acceptance' of homosexuality, prostitution and promiscuity.

AIDS could also bring about enormous changes in how people view sexuality. The notion of safe sex forces us to question many of the assumptions we hold about sex. It demands that we re-evaluate forms of sex that are often considered 'second-best'. It challenges the belief that people, but more especially men, have little voluntary control over their sexual desires (a belief that is frequently reflected in attitudes towards rape, prostitution and porno-graphy). It encourages the development of new meanings for sex and the erotic which are not focused on intercourse, or on necessarily having an orgasm. It could lead to better communication between partners, which may enable women to protect themselves better from other sexual risks such as abusive and unwanted sex. It could enhance intimacy and broaden our enjoyment of sex. If offers an opportunity to talk more openly about sex and to raise issues about sexual choice and control. It could lead to men taking their share of responsibility for making sex safer. It could help break down sexual divisions and stereotypes by emphasising the importance of what you do, rather than how you label yourself. (The recognition that Rock Hudson died of AIDS was shocking; at least partly because it challenged traditional notions of the heterosexual hero and the gay man.) AIDS also challenges what is considered 'natural' or 'normal' about sex. In being advised to practise safer sex we are, in a sense, being urged to be 'unnatural'.

The assumption, very often, is that such changes in sexual attitudes and behaviour will be difficult for most of us. Safe sex will have to be sold to people as fun, exciting and satisfying before they will want to practise it.

This may be more true of men than women. As part of their socialisation, men often come to associate worthwhile sex with intercourse leading to orgasm. One reason, therefore, why men may find it difficult to alter their sexual behaviour in the light of AIDS is that they do not regard safe sex as erotic. Another possible reason is that such changes would represent a threat to their identity and self-esteem. In our society sexual intercourse for men is often a way of achieving status and power over others, and is inextricably linked with being masculine.

There are other reasons why AIDS may be more challenging to male sexuality than to female. With the onset of AIDS many men are experiencing what women have always experienced: an association between sex and danger. Fear of disease is only part of the dangers associated for women with sexuality. Alongside the possibility of sexual pleasure, fear of sexuality is traditionally instilled in women. Fear of being raped. Fear of becoming pregnant. Fear of the health risks associated with using the pill or other forms of contraception. Fear of being humiliated and hurt.

The association of death and desire is also nothing new for women. The physical harm done to victims of sexual violence reminds us of the fatal consequences sex can have for women. The threat of male violence is, however, not the only way in which sex for women has been linked with the possibility of death. Earlier this century it was not uncommon for women to die in childbirth. A woman's fear of sexuality, in this sense, was related to the prospect of repeated pregnancies. Women have also died as a result of trying to abort an unwanted pregnancy, either by their own efforts or at the hands of a back street abortionist.

The idea that there is a consequence to sexual behaviour has also resurfaced with AIDS. During this century most men have not had to think about the consequences of their sexual behaviour in any serious way, while women have always had to do so whether in terms of the risk of pregnancy, health risks associated with contraceptive use, or loss of reputation. Now men are being increasingly forced to consider risk and to take responsibility for their actions – or are they?

It seems that it is taken for granted that women will have to take responsibility for safer sex because men won't. During 'AIDS week', in February 1987, all four TV channels broadcast a series of programmes on AIDS. Time and time again girls were asked if they would carry condoms; boys were asked if they would agree to use them. (The assumption being that men are 'naturally' less able to exercise sexual self-control and are, therefore, less responsible than women.)

This highlights the fact that despite the emphasis in AIDS campaigns to take personal responsibility for our *own* actions, it is women who are frequently responsible for protecting men, as well as themselves, from infection. As the expected gatekeepers of male sexuality, it is they who are landed with the burden of preventing the spread of AIDS, within the heterosexual population at least. Yet ironically, what such a view of heterosexual relationships invariably fails to recognise, is that in a culture where women are expected to be sexually passive, where sex within marriage is legally defined as a man's right, where rape and sexual abuse are primarily crimes against women, many women will have little if any 'choice' whether safer sex occurs or not.

At the same time, the message now being given to girls

and women to carry condoms and encourage their use as part of safer sex raises interesting contradictions. While ignoring practicalities, and the fact that in doing this women are at risk of being labelled an 'easy lay', it challenges the traditional idea that men, not women, should initiate, seek out, and be prepared for sex.

There is also a major contradiction in emphasising the correct use of condoms as the best way of preventing AIDS. You are most at risk of contracting HIV if you engage in anal or vaginal penetration. Yet, despite this, AIDS education campaigns have, by and large, uncritically accepted a view of sex as intercourse. We have the 'condom solution'. Safer sex advice is centred upon fewer sexual partners and being told 'always use a condom'. (Though as a woman I find it difficult to know where I should wear one.) Why do we never hear about non-penetrative sex as a less risky and potentially more pleasurable way of preventing AIDS? Because it's too challenging both to men in general, and to the view of intercourse as 'natural' or 'normal' sex: a view that is enshrined in the law and religious teachings.

To advocate non-penetrative sex would not only transform the meaning of sex from sexual reproduction to sexual pleasure, but also would have positive implications for the majority of women who do not have orgasms through intercourse. It would underline the fact that this is neither abnormal nor a problem, but a valid form of sexual expression. It would also provide an opportunity to discuss lesbian and gay relationships in a more positive light. For instance, when intercourse and penetration are no longer the key words in the language of love, lesbians will hopefully be spared the age-old question 'But what do you *do*?' – which, when translated, means without a penis what can you do?

These are not new issues. Feminists, both earlier this century and more recently, have criticised sexual relationships between men and women, with the emphasis on penetration, as, very often, unsatisfying and dangerous for women. There is consequently a certain irony and not a little anger involved in observing the way in which the government, media and medical profession have responded to the AIDS crisis. It's as if only now, when men's health is at stake, do we need to consider sexual risks and responsibilities. Why wasn't there a campaign for safer sex ten or fifteen years ago? The answer that AIDS is life-threatening is not sufficient. Cervical cancer is the cause of 4,000 deaths every year in British women. Safer sex has a major role to play in the prevention of cervical cancer. Taking birth control pills and other forms of contraceptives can be associated with serious side-effects, which can be fatal. None of these are associated with condom use or non-penetrative sex.

The challenge of AIDS is to create new meanings of sexuality that are not based primarily on heterosexual intercourse, or on men having more control over sexuality than women. Far from being a restrictive influence, we could see this as liberating for women, in terms of their relationships with men. Similarly, the new need to communicate about sex is something which could benefit women. The more women know about their bodies, and about sexuality and reproduction, the more likely they are to be able to take control of what is happening to them.

AIDS could also lead to a 'sexual revolution' that would have very different implications for women. In the United States AIDS has led to the repackaging of sex as a commercial product. Despite AIDS, it's still 'sex for sale'. Telephone sex (where people pay to masturbate whilst talking over the phone to someone else); jack-off-clubs (where men pay to masturbate in front of others); and HIV-antibody negative dating clubs are the massage parlours, bathhouses and singles bars of the nineties. Also, if fantasy be the stuff of safer sex, then it's easy to see how this can be used to defend pornography. Already the pornography industry has begun to market safer sex videos, books and magazines. AIDS also has the potential to lead to further restrictions in women's reproductive rights and, as we have already begun to witness in relation to prostitutes and lesbians, to calls for new forms of social control over sexuality. In this sense, the real challenge of AIDS is to recognise the need for safer sexual practices, while insisting on a much broader political struggle against the way in which the state, the Church, the media, and men regulate women's lives through their control over sexuality and reproduction.

Note on sources

Very little has so far been written about women and AIDS. In researching this book I have therefore often had to make use of material which is not directly concerned with how the disease affects women. Books which are helpful in providing information on AIDS include the following.

AIDS Concerns You: What Every Man and Woman Should Know About AIDS, Jonathan Weber and Annabel Ferriman, Pagoda, 1986.
AIDS, V. G. Daniels, MTP, 1987.
AIDS: The Story of a Disease, John Green and David Miller, Grafton, 1986.
The Management of AIDS Patients, ed. David Miller, Jonathan Weber and John Green, Macmillan, 1986.
Mobilizing Against AIDS, Institute of Medicine, National Academy of Sciences, Harvard University Press, 1986.
Understanding AIDS, Victor Gong, Cambridge University Press, 1985.

Women and Aids

Advice For Life, Chris Norwood, Pantheon Books, 1987.
AIDS: the Women, eds. Ines Rieder and Patricia Ruppelt, Cleis Press, 1988.
Making It: A woman's guide to sex in the age of AIDS, Cindy Patton and Janis Kelly, Firebrand Books, 1987.
The Real Truth about Women and AIDS, Helen Singer Kaplan, Simon and Schuster, 1987.
Women and AIDS Clinical Resource Guide, San Francisco AIDS Foundation, 1987.

Books Which Deal With The Social And Political Aspects

Aids, Africa and Racism, Richard Chirimuuta and Rosalind Chiri-
muuta, 1987.
AIDS and the New Puritanism, Dennis Altman, Pluto Press, 1986.
AIDS: The Deadly Epidemic, Graham Hancock and Enver Carim,
Gollancz, 1986.
AIDS and the Third World, Panos Institute, revised 1987.
And the Band Played On, Randy Shilts, Penguin, 1988.
Blaming Others, Renee Sabatier, Panos, 1988.
Policing Desire, Simon Watney, Comedia, 1987.
Sex and Germs: The Politics of AIDS, Cindy Patton, South End Press,
1985.

Self-help guides, personal accounts and guides to safer sex

AIDS: A Guide to Survival, Peter Tatchell, Gay Men's Press, 1986.
The Complete Guide to Safe Sex, The Institute for Advanced Study of
Human Sexuality, Prevent, 1987.
Epic of Courage, L. Nungesser, South End Press, 1986.
Living with AIDS: A Guide to Survival by People with AIDS, Front-
liners, 1987.
Living with HIV, David Miller, Macmillan, 1987.
Make it Happy, Make it Safe, Jane Cousins-Mills, Penguin, 1988.
Safer Sex, Peter Gordon and Louise Mitchell, Faber and Faber,
1988.
The Screaming Room, Barbara Peabody, Oak Tree Publications,
1986.
When Someone you Love has AIDS, Betty Clare Moffatt, IBS, 1986.

In writing this book, the following journals were an important
source of information: *Annals of International Medicine, New England
Journal of Medicine, American Journal of Medicine, British Medical
Journal, Nature, Science, Journal of the American Medical Association,
Cancer Research, British Journal of Obstetrics and Gynaecology, Community Care, Morbidity and Mortality Weekly Report*, and *Communicable Disease Report*.

Reference was also made to material published by the Health
Education Council, the Terrence Higgins Trust, the Haemophilia
Society and various AIDS organisations both in the United
Kingdom and the United States.

World and United States figures were obtained from the World Health Organisation (Paris) and the Centers for Disease Control (Atlanta, Georgia).

Sources for British figures included the DHSS, the Communicable Diseases Surveillance Centre, the Haemophilia Society, and the Home Office.

Resources List

Useful addresses

The Terrence Higgins Trust
52–54 Gray's Inn Road,
London WC1X 8JU.
Telephone Helpline **01 242 1010**.
3 p.m.–10 p.m. daily.

Has discussion and support group for women working in the AIDS field. Offers help and counselling to people with HIV or AIDS, and their friends and relatives. Also provides an information service for those who are worried about AIDS. Has a drug group.

The Haemophilia Society
123 Westminster Bridge Road,
London SE1 7HR.
Telephone **01 928 2020**.

Offers information and advice for people with haemophilia, their partners, friends and relatives.

Health Education Authority
78 New Oxford Street,
London WC1 1AH.
Telephone **01 631 0930**.

Produces health education booklets on AIDS which can be ordered through the following address:

Health Education Authority
Department A,
Milton Keynes MK1 1TX.

Leaflet on AIDS and related issues can be obtained by ringing the 24 hour service on **0800 555777**.

National AIDS Helpline

A free national telephone information and advice service on AIDS is available. The number is **0800 567123.**
Women counsellors are always available.

Counselling in the following languages is also available:
Cantonese, Tuesday 6 p.m.–10 p.m. on **0800 282446**
Hindi, Gujerati, Punjabi, Bengali and Urdu, Wednesday 6 p.m.–10 p.m. on **0800 282445**
Afro-Caribbean counsellors are on shift on the main number Fridays 6 p.m.–10 p.m.

Further information on AIDS can be obtained by using the **Healthline Telephone Service**. This is a 24 hour service providing recorded information on a number of AIDS-related issues. Telephone **0345 581151.**

Women's Health and Reproductive Rights Information Centre
52–54 Featherstone Street,
London EC1Y 8RT.
Telephone **01 251 6332.**

Provides general information on women and AIDS.

Family Planning Association

27–35 Mortimer Street,
London WC1M 7RJ.
Telephone **01 636 7866.**

6 Windsor Place,
Cardiff CF1 3BX.
Telephone **0222 42766.**

113 University Street,
Belfast BT7 1HP.
Telephone **0232 246937.**

4 Clifton Street,
Glasgow G3 7LA.
Telephone **041 333 9696.**

Regional offices which will provide information on local FPA clinics. Clinics are run through the NHS and don't need a GP referral.

Brook Advisory Centres
233 Tottenham Court Road,
London W1A 9AE.
Telephone **01 580 2991.**

Clinics in various cities – they provide confidential advice on contraception, pregnancy, abortion and emotional and sexual problems for young people.

Black Community AIDS Team (BCAT)
The Landmark,
47 Tulse Hill,
London SW2 2TN.
Telephone **01 671 7611 or 01 671 7612.**

Positively Women
c/o CLASH (Central London Action on Street Health),
The Soho Hospital,
Soho Square,
London W1.
Telephone **01 734 1794**.

A support group for women who are HIV antibody positive or have AIDS. Meets on alternative Thursdays from 6 p.m.–8 p.m.

Frontliners
52–54 Grays Inn Road,
London WC1X 8JU.
Telephone **01 831 0330** in office hours.
Telephone **01 232 1010** 7 p.m.–10 p.m. every day.

Run by and for people with AIDS, provides information, help and support.

Positive Partners
c/o 10 Rathbone Place, London W1.
Telephone **01 249 6068.**

A support group for partners who are HIV positive or have AIDS.

Body Positive
P.O. Box 493,
London W14 0TF.
Telephone **01 373 9124.**

Run by and for people who are HIV antibody positive. Provides support, and help and advice.

SCODA (Standing Conference on Drug Abuse)
1–4 Hatton Place,
London EC1N 8ND.
Telephone **01 430 2341.**

Provides information and advice to drug users on HIV and AIDS, including details of your nearest needle exchange. Has a full list of local services for drug users throughout the country. (During the times SCODA is not operating the Samaritans may be able to provide similar information by consulting the SCODA directory.)

Mainliners
359 Old Kent Road,
London SE1.
Telephone **01 231 1528.**

Run by and for current and ex-drug users who are HIV positive, or have AIDS or other HIV-related illness. They provide help, support and information.

DAWN (Drugs, Alcohol, Women Nationally)
Omnibus Workspace,
39–41 North Road,
London N7 9DP.
Telephone **01 700 4653.**

Provides information, support and advice for women on drug use, and on HIV and AIDS.

London Lesbian and Gay Switchboard
BM Switchboard,
London WC1N 3XX.
Telephone **01 837 7324** (24 hour service).

A telephone advisory and counselling service run by lesbians and gay men. Can answer general queries about AIDS and put you in touch with AIDS organisations and STD clinics.

STD Clinics

STD clinics offer general advice about AIDS and can give you the HIV antibody test. They can also provide counselling for people who have AIDS or are antibody positive, and for their relatives and friends. You can refer yourself to an STD clinic. You don't need a letter from your doctor.

Most clinics are listed in the phone book under Sexually Transmitted Disease or Venereal Disease. Alternatively phone the local hospital, Family Planning Association or the British Pregnancy Advisory Service for the number. The FPA and the BPAS may also be able to provide useful information.

Regional AIDS groups

ENGLAND

Birmingham: AIDS line West Midlands
'Hazeliegh',
79 Stanmore Road,
Edgbaston,
Birmingham B16 9SU.
Telephone **021 622 1511** Monday to Friday 7.30 p.m.–10 p.m. (answerphone at other times).

Bradford: Pennine AIDS Link
P.O. Box 167,
Bradford BD1 1LL.
Telephone **0274 732939**.

Bristol: Alex Richards Trust
1 Mark Lane,
Bristol BS1 4XR.
Telephone **0272 273436**. Monday to Friday 7 p.m.–9 p.m.

Leeds: Leeds AIDS Advice
P.O. Box 172,
Leeds LS7 3B7.
Telephone **0532 444209**. Monday to Friday 8 p.m.–10 p.m.
Office telephone **0532 423204**.

Liverpool: Merseyside AIDS Support Group
63 Shamrock Road,
Birkenhead L41 0EG.
Telephone **051 708 0234.**
Wednesday 7 p.m.–10 p.m.
or **051 246 8089** (recorded message giving details of clinics, AIDS
support, etc.)

Manchester: Manchester AIDS Line
P.O. Box 201,
Manchester M60 1PU.
Telephone **061 228 1617.**
Monday to Friday 7 p.m.–10 p.m. (answerphone at other times.)

Manchester Body Positive
Telephone **061 228 2212.**
Tuesday and Thursday 7.30 p.m.–10 p.m.

Newcastle: AIDS North
Box NE99 1BD,
Newcastle-upon-Tyne.
Telephone **091 232 2855.**
Wednesday and Friday 7 p.m.–10 p.m.
Members of Body Positive on shift Friday 7 p.m.–10 p.m.

Oxford: OXAIDS
Freepost,
The Monument Wing,
The Radclyffe Infirmary,
Woodstock Road,
Oxford OX2 6HE.
Telephone **0865 728817** (office and helpline).
Sunday, Monday, Wednesday and Friday.

Wakefield: Wakefield AIDS Support Group
c/o Department 15,
Clayton Hospital,
Northgate, Wakefield.

WALES

Welsh Health Promotion Authority
Brunel House, No. 2 Fitzalan Road,
Cardiff.

Provides information and advice, and leaflets in English and
Welsh.
Telephone **0222 472472**.

Cardiff AIDS Helpline
Telephone **0222 223433.**
Monday to Friday 7 p.m.–10 p.m.

Gwent
Telephone (Caerlean) **0633 422532.**
Tuesday 2 p.m.–8 p.m.
Telephone (Newport) **0633 841901.**
Monday to Friday 8.30 a.m.–4.30 p.m.

SCOTLAND

Edinburgh and Glasgow: Scottish AIDS Monitor
P.O. Box 169, Edinburgh EH1 3UU.
Telephone (Edinburgh) **031 558 1167.**
Monday to Friday 7.30 p.m.–10 p.m.

Telephone (Glasgow) **041 221 7467.**
Tuesday 7 p.m.–10 p.m.

NORTHERN IRELAND

Belfast: AIDS Belfast
c/o Cara Friend, P.O. Box 44, Belfast BT1 1SH.
Telephone **0232 226117.**
Monday to Friday 7.30 p.m.–10.30 p.m.

UNITED STATES

National AIDS hotlines

(800) 342 AIDS (2437).
Monday to Friday 8.30 a.m.–5.30 p.m.
(800) 634 7477.

Useful National addresses

Centers for Disease Control
1600 Clifton Road, NE,
Atlanta, GA 30333.

The official organisation monitoring the AIDS epidemic in the United States.

Women's AIDS Network
c/o San Francisco AIDS Foundation
333 Valencia Street, 4th Floor,
San Francisco, CA 94103.
Telephone **(415) 864 4376.**

Information exchange, liaison among members in their work with AIDS.

AWARE (Association for Women's AIDS Research and Education)
San Francisco General/Ward 84,
995 Potrero Avenue,
San Francisco, CA 94110.
Telephone **(415) 476 4091.**

Women and AIDS Research Network (WARN)
Washington Square Church,
135 West 4th Street,
New York, NY 10012.
Telephone evenings **(718) 237 2156.**

Provides information on services available for women and children with AIDS. Carers available to assist are welcome.

People with AIDS Coalition
263A West 19th Street,
New York, NY 10011.
Telephone **(212) 627 1810.**

Support and services for people with AIDS and AIDS-related conditions.

Gay Men's Health Crisis
254 West 18th Street,
New York, NY 10011.
Telephone **(212) 807 7035.**

AIDS Hotline: (212) 807 6655.

AUSTRALIA

The Australian Federation of AIDS Organisations
P.O. Box 174, Richmond, Victoria, NSW 3121
Telephone **03 417 1759.**

Australian Capital Territory (ACT)

AIDS Trust of Australia (Canberra)
Telephone **062 47 3993.**

AIDS Information Line **062 57 2855.**

New South Wales

AIDS Council of New South Wales (ACON)
P.O. Box 350, Darlinghurst, NSW 2010.
Telephone **02 211 0499.**

AIDS Hotline **02 332 4000.**
8 a.m.–10 p.m. Monday to Friday.
9 a.m.–6 p.m. Saturday and Sunday.

Lifeline Sydney **02 264 2222** (24 hours).

Lifeline Sydney Youthline **02 264 1177**.
Midday to midnight, 7 days a week.

Ethnicline **008 04 3124.**
10 a.m.–10 p.m. Monday to Friday.
AIDS Trust Of Australia (Sydney)
Telephone **02 211 2161.**

Northern Territory

Northern Territory AIDS Council
Telephone **089 41 1711.**

Crisisline
Telephone **089 81 2040.**
7 p.m.–7 a.m. daily.

Queensland

Queensland (North) AIDS Council
Telephone **07 844 1990.**

Queensland (South) AIDS Council
Telephone **07 721 1384.**

Queensland AIDS Committee
Telephone **07 854 1758** (local calls).
        008 17 7434 (country calls).

South Australia

South Australia AIDS Council
Telephone **08 223 6322.**

South Australia Health Commission AIDS Programme
Telephone **08 218 3668.**
9 a.m.–5 p.m.

Victoria

Victoria AIDS Council
61–63 Rupert Street, Collingwood, Melbourne.
Telephone **03 417 1759.**

AIDS Line **03 419 3166.**
(Country callers reverse charges.)

Western Australia

Western Australia AIDS Council
Telephone **09 227 8355.**

AIDS Helpline (Perth) **09 227 8619.**

Country helpline **008 19 9287.**

Perth AIDS Information and Training
Telephone **09 222 6066.**

Tasmania

Tasmania AIDS Council
Telephone **002 31 1930.**

NEW ZEALAND

New Zealand AIDS Foundation
Box 6663, Wellesley Street, Auckland 1.
NZ 33 124.

Glossary

AIDS   An abbreviation for Acquired Immune Deficiency Syndrome. It is thought to be caused by a virus known as HIV, in which the body's immune system is seriously damaged. As a result people who have AIDS are susceptible to some rare cancers and often fatal infections.

AID   Artificial Insemination by Donor. A simple procedure, by which sperm from a donor is placed in a woman's vagina using a syringe.

Anal intercourse (buggery; sodomy; rectal sex; arse-fucking) Sex where a man puts his penis into another person's rectum.

Antibodies   Chemical substances developed by the immune system to fight infectious agents found in the body.

Antibody positive   A blood test result showing that the person has been infected with HIV at some time and developed antibodies to it. It does *not* mean a person has AIDS.

Anus   The opening at the lower end of the bowel.

ARC   Stands for AIDS-related complex. People with ARC have some symptoms associated with HIV infection but do not have any of the opportunistic infections and cancers associated with the diagnosis of AIDS. A proportion of people with ARC go on to develop AIDS.

Bisexual   a woman or man who desires sexual relationships with both sexes.

Caesarean birth   A method of childbirth in which a surgical incision is made through the abdominal wall and uterus.

Cervix   The neck of the uterus or womb.

Clitoris ('clit')   A small, complex organ located where the inside-lips of the vagina meet. It plays an important role in a woman's orgasm.

Clitoridectomy   The surgical removal of the clitoris and the inner and sometimes outer lips of the vagina.

Condom (sheath; rubber; johnny)   A thin rubber sheath worn over a man's penis to reduce the risk of pregnancy, venereal disease, or infection with HIV.

Cunnilingus (oral sex; licking; go down on; sucking)   When a person uses their tongue or mouth to stimulate a woman's genitals.

Diaphragm   A round latex object inserted in the vagina to cover the cervix. Used as a contraceptive method.

Ejaculation   Discharge of semen (cum) from a man's penis.

Erection (hard on)   The engorgement of the penis with blood.

Factor 8   An ingredient in the blood which is needed for the blood to clot normally.

Faeces   Waste products; excrement; shit. 'Scat' is a slang term for sexual activities that involve faeces.

Fellatio (cock-sucking; blow job; giving head; go down on; oral sex)   When a person uses their tongue or mouth to stimulate a man's penis.

Fisting (fist-fucking; hand-balling)   This is where someone inserts their entire hand into another person's vagina or rectum.

French (wet) kiss   A kiss that includes tongue contact and exchange of saliva (spit).

Gay   A man or woman who finds others of the same gender sexually attractive and defines himself or herself as such (see also Homosexual; Lesbian).

Genitalia   The external sex organs. In women this area is called the vulva and includes the inner and outer lips (labia) of the vagina, and the clitoris. In men this term refers to the penis, the scrotum and testicles (balls; nuts).

Gonorrhoea (clap; a dose)   A sexually transmitted disease caused by bacteria.

Haemophilia   A rare disease of the blood which mainly affects men. People with haemophilia need treatment to help their blood to clot (see also Factor 8).

Hand-to-genital sex (e.g. mutual masturbation; to wank someone off; hand job; finger-fucking)   Where a person uses their hand or fingers to stimulate their partner's genitals.

Herpes   A viral infection that produces painful blisters usually in the mouth or genital area, and can be transmitted during sex.

Heterosexual ('straight')   A term used to describe sexual relationships between women and men.

HIV Stands for human immunodeficiency virus. HIV is the name researchers have agreed upon for the virus which causes AIDS (see also HTLV-3; LAV).

HIV antibody test A blood test which shows whether or not a person has antibodies to the virus which causes AIDS. The test indicates only whether a person has at some time been infected with HIV. It cannot determine if a person has AIDS or will develop AIDS in future.

Homophobia This is often used to describe fear/hatred/discrimination against gay men. Its equivalent against women is anti-lesbianism.

Homosexual (gay) Used to describe sex between two men and, to a lesser extent, two women. Also used to describe a *person* as homosexual or gay (see also Gay; Lesbian).

HTLV-3 or Human T-cell Lymphotropic Virus Type-3 The name American researchers first gave to the virus which causes AIDS.

Immune System The system in the body which fights infection.

Infibulation A form of clitoridectomy where the two sides of the vulva are sewn up after the clitoris has been removed.

Injecting drug user A person who injects drugs.

Intercourse (fucking; screwing; penetration; having sex) When a man puts his penis into a woman's vagina this is called vaginal intercourse. When he puts it into a person's rectum (back passage) this is called anal intercourse.

IUD Stands for intra-uterine device. A small plastic object which can be inserted into a woman's womb to prevent pregnancy.

IV An abbreviation for intravenous. It is often used to describe drug users who inject drugs directly into their veins.

KS An abbreviation for Kaposi's sarcoma, a rare form of skin cancer which people with AIDS often get.

KY The brand name for a water-based lubricant for sex.

LAV Lymphadenopathy associated virus, the name French researchers first gave to the virus causing AIDS.

Lesbian (dyke; lezzie; gay) A woman who finds other women sexually attractive and defines herself as such.

Lymphadenopathy A chronic condition of swollen lymph nodes.

Menstrual blood Blood that is shed from a woman's uterus during her period.

Monogamous Having sex with only one person.

Nonoxynol-9   A chemical agent in some spermicides and lubricants, which may reduce the risk of infection with HIV.

Opportunistic infections   Infections which take advantage of the opportunity offered by the body's weakened immune system to cause illness.

Oral sex   (see Cunnilingus; Fellatio).

Oral-anal sex (analingus; rimming)   Where a person uses their mouth or tongue to stimulate another person's anus (arsehole; bumhole).

PCP   An abbreviation of pneumocystis carinii pneumonia. An infection of the lungs, this is a common illness in people with AIDS.

Penis (cock; dick; willie; prick; shaft)   The male sex organ, also used for urination (peeing).

PGL   Stands for persistent generalised lymphadenopathy. This refers to a group of people who have persistently enlarged lymph glands, but who do not have any other symptoms of HIV infection. A proportion of people with PGL go on to develop AIDS.

PWA   An abbreviation for people with AIDS.

Rectum (back passage)   This is the lower part of the bowel, ending in the anus (arsehole; bumhole).

Safer sex   Sex which reduces the risk of infection with HIV, unwanted pregnancy and sexually transmitted diseases.

Sado-masochism (S/M)   When erotic enjoyment is obtained through giving or receiving physical or psychological pain.

Saliva (spit)   The clear water like fluid found in the mouth.

Semen (cum)   Fluid ejaculated from a man's penis.

Sero-positive   A person who has antibodies to HIV (see Antibody positive).

SI or self-insemination   The term used when a woman carries out artificial insemination without the help of doctors or an official donor organisation.

Special clinic (see STD clinic).

Spermicide   A chemical substance that kills sperm.

STDs   (see also VD) An abbreviation for sexually transmitted diseases.

STD clinic (VD clinic; genito-urinary clinic)   A clinic which specialises in dealing with sexually transmitted diseases.

T cells   A group of white blood cells that protect the body against foreign agents, but which may be rendered ineffective by HIV.

Urethra　The tube which conducts the urine from the bladder out of the body.

Urine　(wee, piss; pee).

Vaccine　A sustance that causes immunity to a disease.

Vagina (cunt)　The organ in women leading from the vulva to the uterus or womb.

Vaginal intercourse　(fucking; screwing; penetration; having sex; copulation; coitus) Sex where a man puts his penis into a woman's vagina.

VD　Abbreviation for venereal disease. Any of a range of diseases that may be transmitted through sexual intercourse.

Virus　Extremely small micro-organisms which cause many diseases.

Vulva　External sex organs in women; includes the outer and inner lips of the vagina and the clitoris.

Watersports (or golden showers)　Slang term for sexual activities that involve urine.

Works　A term used by drug users to refer to equipment used for mixing or injecting drugs.

Index